The Guide to
Great Sex

How to Get Better in Bed and Take
Your Sex Life to the Next Level

Michael Karp

DISCLAIMER (DO NOT SKIP THIS)

I am not a doctor, sex therapist, or trained professional in sexual health. I am a former sex columnist who took it upon himself to read and learn as much as he could about sex and sexuality and who seeks fulfillment in his sex life by practicing this knowledge.

The advice given in this book is a mixture of research I have done, my personal experience, and my unique view on this aspect of life. It is a *guide*, meaning that it is up to you to decide whether some or all of this information should be applied to your own sex life. I truly believe that this book can help anyone achieve better sex, no matter how much experience they have. But I am not a professional, and will not be held accountable for any adverse outcomes of practicing what I have written here.

In the end, you are the final decision maker, and you hold total responsibility in your sex life.

Legal Notice

This guide assumes that all readers are, or will be, participating in legal and consensual sexual activity, and the examples are presented under the same assumption. The Purchaser or Reader of this publication assumes responsibility for the use of these materials and information. Adherence to all applicable laws and regulations, federal, state, and local, or any other jurisdiction is the sole responsibility of the Purchaser or Reader. The Author and Publisher assume no responsibility or liability whatsoever on the behalf of any Purchaser or Reader of these materials.

Copyright © Michael Karp, 2015. All Rights Reserved.

No part of this publication may be reproduced or transmitted in any form or by any means, mechanical or electronic, including photocopying and recording, or by any information storage and retrieval system, without permission in writing from the publisher.

With that out of the way, enjoy the rest of the book.

ISBN-13: 978-1-5218-6914-7

Table of Contents

GLOSSARY 1
PREFACE 4
Chapter 1 MY STORY 7
Chapter 2 WHAT IS GREAT SEX? 13
Chapter 3 UNDERSTANDING THE INTRICACIES OF PLEASURE AND ORGASMS 16
Chapter 4 FOREPLAY: HOW TO TEASE YOUR PARTNER AND HEIGHTEN SEXUAL AROUSAL 23
Chapter 5 ORAL SEX: FELLATIO AND CUNNILINGUS TECHNIQUES 36
Chapter 6 ANAL SEX 53
Chapter 7 16 POWERFUL POSITIONS FOR THE HOTTEST SEX AND DEEPEST INTIMACY 59
Chapter 8 HOW SEX TOYS CAN IMPROVE YOUR SEX LIFE 75
Chapter 9 GETTING VOCAL IN THE BEDROOM - A SIMPLE ACT THAT CAN TAKE YOUR SEX LIFE TO THE NEXT LEVEL 84
Chapter 10 THE ART OF THE TRANSITION 93
Chapter 11 DEVELOPING SEXUAL INTUITION 107
Chapter 12 MASTERING MULTITASKING 111
Chapter 13 THE BALANCE OF DOMINANCE 120
Chapter 14 COMMUNICATION PRACTICES 126
Chapter 15 UNLOCKING SEXUAL FANTASIES AND FETISHES 140
Chapter 16 OVERCOMING SEXUAL ANXIETY AND INSECURITY ... 148
Chapter 17 WHAT ARE YOUR SEXUAL VALUES? 172
Chapter 18 SEXUAL COMPATIBILITY 178
Chapter 19 A NOTE ABOUT PORN 180
Chapter 20 THE SEXUAL CONQUEST 182
REFERENCES and FURTHER READING 184

The Guide to Great Sex

GLOSSARY

Refer to these definitions whenever certain terms become confusing or unclear

Partner – For the purposes of this book: Sexual or romantic partners relating to casual sexual relationships, one-night stands, committed relationships, or any sexual partnership between two human beings.

Stimulation – Any deliberate action done with the purpose of providing pleasure.

Fellatio – Oral stimulation of the penis (Merriam-Webster).

Cunnilingus – Oral stimulation of the vulva or clitoris (Merriam-Webster).

Vagina – The passage leading from the uterus to the vulva (Dictionary.com).

Vulva – The external genitals of those with a vagina, including the outer/inner lips, vaginal entrance, and clitoris.

Clitoris – A small erectile organ at the anterior or ventral part of the vulva homologous to the penis (Merriam-Webster). A ball of tissue located at the north end of the vulva where the lips come together. Typically said to be the epicenter of all pleasure for people who have vaginas.

Clitoral Shaft – "Attached to the head, and running just beneath the surface of the skin, the clitoral shaft can be easily felt, especially when aroused and filled with blood. A soft little pipe, the shaft is composed of spongy erectile tissue that is extremely receptive to sensation" (*She Comes First*, Ian Kerner, Ph. D.) Area above the head of the clitoris.

Inner/Outer Lips – The labia minora and labia majora of the vulva. Become engorged with blood during arousal and are sensitive to stimulation.

Vaginal Entrance – Entrance to the vagina from the vulva, filled with pleasurable nerve endings.

G-Spot – A cluster of nerve endings located on the roof about 2 inches into the vagina. Often said to be a part of the clitoral network (related to the clitoris in providing pleasure.)

Clitoral Crura – Two "legs" of the clitoral network which extend down both sides of the inner part of the vagina. Said to be related to clitoral, vaginal, and anal stimulation.

Perineum – Area of skin between the genitals and anus. Responds pleasurably to massage as it contains nerves that correlate directly to both the penis and the vagina/vulva.

Penis – Reproductive organ consisting of a shaft, head, and testicles.

Head of the penis – Sensitive mass of tissue that forms the tip of the penis.

Shaft – The main body of the penis.

Testicles – Two organs located in a sack below the penis.

Prostate – A gland responsible for the production of fluid which adds to semen. Contains nerve endings which make it pleasurable when stimulated. It is analogous to the nerve ending cluster of the G-Spot.

The Art of the Transition – Deliberate transition from one move to another in relation to one's sexual flow.

Sexual Intuition – When you instinctively know what you want to do next in the bedroom and how to do it. An understanding of what is happening between the sheets as it happens in real time.

Multitasking – Adding in subtle pleasurable acts that lead to huge differences in the bedroom. Combining these acts with another sexual activity, usually involving the stimulation of the genitals.

The Balance of Dominance/Submission – Balance between the dominant and submissive characteristics of both partners. Relates to each other's sexual tendencies.

Sexual Values – What one values in the bedroom in relation to the standards they hold themselves to and what they value in sexual partners. Examples are communication, safety, trust, comfort, etc.

Sexual Compatibility – How well two people match together on a sexual level. How well your sexual desires, biology, and values fit together with your partner. Can be something you intuitively feel, but it can also be raised and nurtured.

Michael Karp

PREFACE

If you're like me, you grew up hearing things like, "Wait until you are married to have sex" or "Sex only happens between two people who love each other" or "Here are all the terrible consequences of having sex: STI's, unwanted pregnancy, rape, etc."

I don't know about you, but growing up learning about sex this way gave me a pretty jaded view of the entire act. It made me ashamed to express my sexual desire and to see myself as a sexual person. In a society that markets sex *everywhere*, and with peers talking about it constantly, it became a frustrating area of my life.

Luckily, I went to a university with an open sexual environment. I made supportive friends who helped me see the bright side of sex I had never been introduced to before. Eventually, in my final semester, I became the the University newspaper's sex columnist.

I studied sex as much as, if not more than, my major for the entire semester. I began understanding how to make it a more positive aspect of my life, instead of an area that caused me stress and anxiety.

I created this guide to help other people achieve the same thing. I believe that sex is a fundamental need of human beings, and that this need lies on a physical, emotional, and spiritual level.

It's important stuff.

I'm assuming that if you are reading this guide, it's important to you too.

This guide is a combination of what I have read, what I have learned, and what I have experienced as I navigated and continue to navigate the sexual unknown.

What will we be discussing here? I am going to explain everything I know about living a healthy sex life and how to achieve it yourself:

We'll be talking about foreplay, oral sex, understanding how pleasure works, orgasms, positions that provide the most exhilarating sensations, sex toys, understanding the flow of sexual intercourse, multitasking, domination, and much, much more to give you the knowledge you need to have the best sex you possibly can.

This book is entirely gender and sexual orientation neutral. I have put a vast amount of effort into orienting the book this way. I believe this information is applicable to everyone no matter who they are, and I also believe that everyone deserves to have great sex.

As a result of this, you may read sentences that are phrased awkwardly, such as, "…those with a [insert body part here]" instead of a gender being stated. You will also see me use the word "partner" a fair amount.

Let's define it quickly. For the purposes of this book, "partner" refers to…

"Sexual or romantic partners relating to casual sexual relationships, one-night stands, committed relationships, or any sexual partnership between two human beings."

I may phrase ideas and examples in a way that seems like I'm only discussing a certain type of relationship. Unless I explicitly state it, assume I am using the definition above.

Sounds good? Sweet deal.

Excited? Me too.

So, without further ado, let's get started.

Chapter 1

MY STORY

First, a little bit about me and my sexual history. I want you to get a feel for where I'm coming from and how I ended up writing this book.

I lost my virginity when I was 18. It was about halfway through my freshman year of college. Before this, I had a whopping TWO sexual experiences under my belt. I know. Playa playa.

There is a part of me that wishes I had lost it sooner, because it was a huge relief getting it out of the way and having its weight lifted off my shoulders. I know your first time is "supposed" to be awesome, but how many people do you know that actually had a good first time?

There *is* a reason why I don't regret it. It was around 1:30 AM after I lost my virginity, so naturally I texted my best bud and told him about it (who happened to be a virgin at the time). The exchange went something like this:

"Dude guess what!? I just lost my virginity!"

"No way! Now I'm the last one of the three of us!" (the three best friends from childhood).

About 2 hours later he texted me saying he had lost his virginity as well.

How many people can say they lost their virginity on the same night as their best friend? Not many, I'm guessing. That's too cool to regret. Now we have an excuse to party for the rest of our lives. The annual virginniversary!

Over the next 7 months or so, I had some random, few yet far between, and not-so-fulfilling sexual experiences. We can list whiskey dick (too drunk to get it up) among the highlights of those experiences.

It wasn't until I got my first sex buddy (non-committed sexual partner) my sophomore year that I gained any sort of confidence or useful experience in the bedroom.

When you first start having sex, there is a part of you that needs to validate how you've been imagining yourself in bed all this time. Can you actually do what you've seen in porn and/or movies? Is that what it is really like? Can I even pleasure this person?

That's a lot of uncertainty for an act that's supposed to be this fiery, passionate connection and an explosion of pleasure and emotion.

Luckily, I was with a partner who was more experienced than me and supported me as I figured things out.

I'm sure many people go through something like this in the beginning, whether it is in a committed relationship, a casual sexual relationship, or numerous casual relationships. There is an initial growth period.

After this growth period, I sort of hit a plateau. I went through periods where I was having a lot of sex and periods where I was in a sexual funk.

In all honesty, as many people that age do, I placed too much of my identity and self-worth on how much sex I was having and who I was having it with.

It's an unhealthy place to be and a poor mindset for achieving happiness in any area of your life. Of course, I didn't know this then, so rollercoasters of anxiety and bliss followed.

I came into my own around the end of junior year. I stopped caring about whether I was having sex, who I was having it with, and what other people thought of me. I focused all of my efforts on simply having as much fun as possible.

Ironically, but not coincidentally, this is when I started having some of the best sex of my life with partners I actually cared about and enjoyed being around. Little did I know, this was a BIG step towards having great sex.

The culminating point came about a quarter of the way into my senior year. I got a girlfriend — my first serious relationship in 4 years. I was a virgin back then, but I was not a virgin now.

I discovered that I enjoy sober sex WAY more than drunk sex. I had experienced sober sex before this, but it was usually after a night of partying and with alcohol still affecting me.

Sober sex is raw. It's real. There's nothing clouding your thoughts or putting you on autopilot. The emotions are felt to their fullest, the pleasure is felt to its fullest, and everything is laid barren before you.

That is real sex.

I've always loved talking about sex. Communication has never been an issue for me. But communicating with someone you've given your full self to, emotionally and sexually, manifests itself in your sex life in ways you could have never imagined.

The spark that lit the flame:

"Hey. Why don't we just get really good at sex?"

I said that to my girlfriend somewhere near the beginning of our relationship, and it began a journey into kama sutra, positions, toys, dominance, public sex, and eventually, a writing gig.

Huh? Whatchu talking 'bout, Willis?

As my buddy and I were walking back from class one day and he picked up a copy of the school newspaper. On the back, it listed openings for the next semester. He noticed that the sex columnist position was opening up, and decided to joke around by telling me I should apply.

I decided I had nothing to lose, so I applied, sent in a writing sample, got an interview, and to my surprise, they called me the next day and told me I got the position.

I ended up producing over 28 articles that semester. It was a great experience in growth, humility, vulnerability, and sexual knowledge that I will never forget.

The guide you're reading right now is rooted in the knowledge I gained during that semester — reading books, studies, doing interviews (okay, just one interview. I'm not a journalist), and pushing my physical and mental limits in the bedroom.

Reading that last sentence, it sounds like I was obsessed with this stuff. You could call it an obsession, but it was an obsession in growth and seeing just how far I could delve into this topic that had eluded me for so many years.

Yes, I overcompensated. But now I am writing about it to help other people improve their own sex lives. I think that is beyond worth it.

I have since branched off from sex into other absurdly healthy obsessions, such as writing and building an online business. But I still love having sex, I still love trying new things, and I still love writing about it.

At its core, sex is about receiving pleasure, giving pleasure, building connections, expressing feelings, having fun, and enjoying the thrill of sexual exploration.

However, everyone experiences sex differently. We each have a unique viewpoint on what determines the quality of our sexual experiences.

This book is meant as a guide to help you find that unique viewpoint. Although I fully believe in the words written here, I don't believe that you should take everything as a matter of fact.

I want you to take this information and use it to find your own way through the sexual world, to find the truth behind *your* sexuality and what it means in your own life, and to utilize it in maximizing the experiences you have with each sexual partner, as each partner is a unique journey and exploration in their own right.

I've mentioned great sex a couple times. This *is* called *The Guide to Great Sex,* after all.

It's time to answer the question:

What the hell is it?

Chapter 2

WHAT IS GREAT SEX?

Truly great sex is an entirely selfless act. You are not having sex just to get laid or to get yourself off. Both people take an interest in each other's pleasure.

But how do you know what pleases each other?

The name of the game is knowledge and communication.

I know. Sexy stuff.

Don't worry, we'll get to the tips and tricks, but for now, it's important to lay this framework.

Great sex happens between two people (and sometimes more) who are great in bed *together*, not just individually. They openly talk about sex with each other:

If they like something, they say it. If they don't like something, they say that as well. They don't waste valuable time they could be spending pleasing each other.

They also work through each other's sexual anxieties and insecurities.

Everyone has some form of sexual anxiety and insecurity, and it is different for every person. Whether you are having sex with someone for one night or for a lifetime, they will come up. It's crucial to be supportive and understanding and to work through it together.

Let each other know there is no judgment, that these things cannot be controlled, and that it's more important to feel comfortable with each other than to avoid it.

We'll be going through anxieties and insecurities in detail in a later chapter, but be aware that even if you don't deal with any yourself, your partner may struggle with them. Handle any that arise in mature manner so you can both ***progress*** within your sex life rather than remain hindered by it.

I've also noticed something that I call "sexual intuition." It develops as you have more sex and learn more about what you're doing. Sexual intuition is an understanding of what is happening between the sheets as it happens in real time.

You can *feel* whether a position is working or not. You can *feel* when your partner is about to have an orgasm and what you need to do to get them there. You *know* that if you do certain things, your partner will love them.

This intuition comes from two things: Having sex and learning about sex.

For most people, it arises naturally as they gain more experience. Fortunately, you can expedite the process by taking an active interest in your sex life and learning as much as you can.

If you want to improve your sex life, you have to take an active interest in it. By active, I mean scouring the internet for information, reading studies on sexual behavior, and reading books like this one to further your understanding and apply that knowledge in the bedroom.

You have undoubtedly heard that knowledge is power.

In this case, knowledge is great sex.

Chapter 3

UNDERSTANDING THE INTRICACIES OF PLEASURE AND ORGASMS

What is pleasure, in its simplest form?

It's the enjoyable feeling of satisfaction you receive when a desire is fulfilled.

When you've been craving a slice of pizza all day, and you get off work, head straight to Pizza Hut, wait patiently for your order to finish, and take that first cheesy, meaty, greasy, glorious bite, THAT feeling right there is pleasure.

Psychology describes pleasure in terms of positive feedback. We are motivated to seek out what gives us pleasure and recreate those instances that have given us pleasure in the past.

For our purposes, first we need to understand pleasure in its physical form (although, its mental form is just as important, and we will see how the two cooperate).

Physical pleasure stems from our central nervous system, the network of neurons that transmit information from all parts of our bodies to our brains.

Nerve endings near the surface of our skin receive these signals first. The density of these nerve endings differ in various parts of our body.

Can you guess where one of the highest concentrations might be?

If you guessed your genitals, you just won the $1 million prize. Well, maybe just a million orgasms (I'd rather have the latter).

According to Ian Kerner, Ph. D., sex counselor, and best-selling author of *She Comes First: The Thinking Man's Guide to Pleasuring a Woman*, the penis contains about 4,000 nerve endings while the clitoris contains about 8,000 (he doesn't note how many in the whole vagina/vulva, but there are more in the outer lips, inner lips, vaginal entrance, and inside the vagina).

That's A LOT. It's no wonder these areas are so sensitive.

You may be thinking, "Alright cool, I'll just focus on mine and my partner's genitals the whole time and we will have amazing orgasms. That's what I figured anyway."

It's not that simple, or that boring. Sexual pleasure is complex, but that is what makes it such an exciting journey to navigate.

I prefer to think less in terms of having sex with my partner's body, and more in terms of having sex with their brain and their mind as well.

I know that sounds strange, but it makes sense considering the brain is where all of our pleasure signals end up.

Breaking Down Orgasms

The road to orgasm is navigated in terms of phases, with mental and physical pleasure playing a part throughout.

Sex researchers, Masters and Johnson, identified four stages to what they call the "sexual response cycle." These stages are Excitement, Plateau, Orgasm, and Resolution.

The following derives from WebMD, sprinkled with my take on each phase.

Stage 1 – Excitement (time frame: A few minutes to several hours)

This is when your body and mind recognize that sexual tension is present.

There are palpable sexual overtones, like when you are dancing with someone at a club, or holding hands walking home together, or lying in bed kissing and rubbing each other.

At this point, muscle tension increases. Sometimes you are not consciously aware of it, but your stomach may have tightened or your leg muscles may have stiffened up.

Your heart rate increases and your breathing becomes deeper.

WebMD states that your skin may become flushed, as in reddish blotches around the chest and back. (I have read this before, but I have never seen or noticed it. I have felt my skin getting warmer, however.)

The nipples harden (woot woot!).

Here's the big one: Blood flow to the genitals increases. The penis becomes erect and the clitoris/inner lips swell. Vaginal lubrication also begins (the vulva, or outer area of the vagina including the lips, clitoris, and vaginal entrance, gets "wet").

Breasts gain in size and the internal vaginal walls start to swell. Testicles also swell, the scrotum tightens, and fluid may secrete from the penis.

Phew!

Now that we're all excited, let's move on to Stage 2.

Stage 2 – Plateau

The plateau is everything from initial stimulation to the moment just before release, or orgasm.

You can view this whole process as a constant buildup of sexual tension, through teasing, give and take, multitasking, and some of the other techniques we'll discuss later which make up the meat of this guide.

In this phase, all of the changes that started in the Excitement phase increase in intensity.

The vulva swells further as blood flow increases. The clitoris becomes more sensitive, and may retract under the clitoral hood if it is overstimulated.

The testicles withdraw into the scrotum, and the penis reaches its maximum erection.

Your breathing, heart rate, and blood pressure increase. (What's interesting to note is that this happens even if the person isn't doing any physical activity during sex. I find that to be strong biological evidence for this part of the response cycle).

Muscle spasms may start to occur in places like the feet, face, hands, and thighs. Muscle tension increases further as well.

Stage 3 – Orgasm

The Big O. The Grand Finale. The Whole Shebang. The Thing We All Live For.

Ooorrrgaasmm.

It's when all of that built up tension and desire is released in one (and sometimes multiple) wave of intense feeling and pleasure. Hormones and endorphins flood the brain in a way that can only be described as pure ecstasy.

It's. Awesome.

And it's awesome giving it to someone else as well, but we'll get to that later.

What happens when we have an orgasm?

Involuntary muscle contractions begin, sometimes quite violently. Heart rate, blood pressure, and breathing reach their peak of intensity.

Muscles in the vagina contract, and the uterus also begins to contract.

Muscles contract at the base of the penis stimulating the ejaculation of semen.

Neurohormones (oxytocin and prolactin) are released, which are largely attributed to our feelings of intense pleasure when we have an orgasm. Endorphins are also released, contributing to the same result.

A reddish flush may appear all over the body, especially in the face.

Stage 4 — Resolution

Resolution is the comedown after climax. It's when your body's responses return back to their pre-excitement phase – i.e. back to normal.

It's also when you get that "Ahhhhh…" feeling of relaxation. Your muscles feel like jello, they are just tired enough to be fatigued, and you may feel heightened intimacy with your partner.

The ***refractory period*** also kicks in at this point. This is the period between the most recent orgasm and when the individual is physically capable of having another one or continuing stimulation.

It's a period where the person needs to rest and recuperate before they can continue more sexual activity.

This period differs for everyone, and even on a circumstantial basis and/or with age, but it is commonly an extended period of time for partners who have a penis. Ever heard partners of those who have a penis complain that their partner falls asleep or can't continue after having an orgasm? The refractory period plays a part in this.

It's important to note that everyone goes through these phases differently and feels them to varying degrees. While there may be a general framework for how everyone progresses to orgasm, we all feel physical pleasure differently, just how people gain pleasure from other things differently, such as pizza.

(I personally don't gain any pleasure from mushrooms. Italian sausage on the other hand…..wait a second. I'll be right back).

That's why communication about what each other likes is so important. It's also why different partners require, and offer a chance at, unique ways to bring them to the highest heights of pleasure.

You also feel pleasure differently than any partners your current partner may have had, so don't forget to tell them what works best for you as well.

As you may have noticed, the physical *responses* described in the sexual response cycle are largely involuntary. But they are just that – responses to the *stimulation* of an external force, whether you are stimulating yourself or someone else is stimulating you, and vice versa.

While specific pleasure responses are far from universal, there are MANY aspects of sex that can be applied to any situation.

This book is largely based on the techniques people can use to confidently find the right combination of sexual vehicles that will lead to great sex.

Great sex with most, if not any partner.

On to the meat of this guide: The need-to-knows of foreplay, oral sex, anal sex, powerful sex positions, sex toys, and dirty talk.

This portion of the guide is quite detailed. If you start to feel overwhelmed, read through it slowly, note the important points, and refer to it later when your mind has given the information a chance to sink in.

Chapter 4

FOREPLAY: HOW TO TEASE YOUR PARTNER AND HEIGHTEN SEXUAL AROUSAL

You may have heard this phrase about foreplay before. It goes something like, "Foreplay begins 24 hours before sex even happens."

What they mean is, foreplay doesn't just encompass the physical stuff right before sex, but also sending sexy texts, naked photos, getting physical with each other, and teasing each other over the course of the day as well.

Here's my take on this:

It's largely BS and only partially true. But the part that's true is very important.

We can go ahead and throw out the whole 24 hours thing. It's a ridiculous expectation for anyone to uphold.

Imagine actually planning to have sex on a certain night, then backtracking 24 hours and saying, "Okay, we're going to start foreplay riiiiight then. You better send me a naked photo or our sex is ruined."

While my example is exaggerated, you shouldn't be looking at foreplay as something that is planned.

Try to cultivate natural sexuality with your partner so that you don't have to be "ready" or force yourself to send sexy texts or anything like that.

Natural sexuality that permeates the whole relationship makes it more spontaneous. It doesn't matter which type of sexual partner you are with, committed or uncommitted. It still applies.

When this happens, you will send sexy photos when you are inspired to, you will tease and touch each other when you are inspired to, and foreplay (in the sense the above phrase is talking about) will have no true beginning because it is always happening.

That being said, I am going to concern you with a specific type of foreplay, because it's the most actionable.

We're going to discuss the foreplay that happens right before sex, when you're in between the sheets and things are getting hot and heavy.

One Assumption...

Let's assume things are being taken slowly. In this case, it's not the stagger into the bedroom, rip each other's clothes off, and "get right into it" sex you see most often in television and movies.

We're talking about the casually walk into the room together, lie in bed next to each other, start kissing, and "see where things go from here" kind of sex.

I'm going to break down specific actions and steps. In no way do I expect anyone to follow these exactly. You would have to have a piece of paper in front of you and check it every couple minutes. I don't expect you to do this.

I *am* expecting that you will get a solid picture in your mind of what is happening, and when you're in the moment, your subconscious will recall what you read here and you will be able to put it into action.

It should also spark ideas of different things you can try, and give you a general overview of how to approach the all-important, often-debated, sexual foreplay.

Foreplay in Action (The Power of Touch)

Finally, foreplay begins. What do you do?

As you are lying next to each other, start kissing and making out. Get sensual with your kisses in the beginning.

Nibble on your partner's tongue and lips. Just barely graze their lips with yours every once in a while, rather than putting on full pressure.

Tease them. Make them want more.

Make them want a full kiss, but don't give it to them just yet.

This is a common theme that you will notice as we go through this book: constantly building up sexual tension (before reaching orgasm).

If you have ever had this done to you, you know how powerful it is and how it elevates your arousal. For simplicity's sake, we can call it "give and take." You are giving stimulation for an amount of time, then you're taking it away before giving it back to them again. It drives your partner crazy, but in a good way.

Continuing on with your foreplay, don't stop kissing. Start touching your partner's body with your hands and legs at the same time. Caress up and down the expanse of their body as you're kissing them. You're slowly heating up the cauldron of desire and arousal.

Remember, you're having sex with your partner's body *and* mind. Touch their body in a way that stimulates their brain and builds up sexual tension.

Yes, you can go straight for the genitals if you want to. But in general, it's not as sexy and doesn't fill up the cauldron of desire like we want it to.

This would be different if we were discussing "stagger into the room" sex. In that case, foreplay is pretty straight forward (you would skip down to where you start touching each other's genitals).

Tease your partner. Move your hands across their body, just barely missing their private parts.

After a short while, simply graze over their genitals, barely touching them enough for your partner to feel it, but not enough for it to be obvious. Send their brain a quick sexual signal.

Then completely stop moving your hands. Keep them in one spot, making them crave your touch again.

After a short while, when you're ready, resume caressing their body.

You are constantly giving stimulation, then taking it away. And each time you give it back, you increase the level of stimulation.

6 key areas to focus on and how to touch them:

- **Under part of the forearm**. This area is very sensitive. Lightly trailing your nails along the under part of your partner's forearms will send tantalizing shivers down your their spine.

- **The sides of their neck and ears**. Placing your hand on this area gives the interaction a romantic vibe. The ears are also pleasure centers, so try gently massaging them, especially the earlobes.

- **Their legs**, especially the calves and feet. Give them a light massage.

- **Their back**. Switch from trailing your fingers down to giving it a good scratch, stopping just above their butt as if you were going to touch it, then moving back up.

- **Their hands**. Every once in a while, grab your partner's hand and interlock fingers. It's romantic and will get the love hormones flowing, increasing sexual desire and intimacy. Even if you're in a casual relationship or it's one-night stand, you can simulate these emotions by doing these actions, increasing the depth of your connection.

- **The hips**. Periodically grab them and pull them towards you, using your thigh to rub against their crotch.

Notice that you haven't directly touched each other's genitals yet, but the tension has built up *so much* that you two almost can't take it anymore.

This pattern of a buildup of tension —> then satisfaction —> buildup —> then satisfaction, plays out the whole way until sex is over. Most of it is subtle, but it leads to noticeable changes in the overall experience.

Going For the Genitals

You've been lightly grazing your partner's genitals everyone once in a while, sending provocative signals to their brain that have caused their body to begin rushing blood to their sexually vital areas (as when blood rushes to the genitals during the Excitement stage).

Don't forget that you are also still kissing each other and making out throughout foreplay.

It's time to take things to the next level.

Make a confident and deliberate move for each other's genitals. No second guessing. No hesitation. It's time for the next phase and you two are ready to go.

If your partner hesitates a bit, you can try taking their hand and gently nudging it towards your genitals, or even placing it right on them.

However, as with any part of the sexual journey, if one of you doesn't feel comfortable or wants to stop, the other must grant that wish and be supportive.

Talk about what made them uncomfortable, see if you two can adjust something, and maybe try again later or another time. But trying to coerce someone into continuing against their will is immoral, borderline unlawful, and sometimes extremely unlawful.

By going for their genitals, I mean purposeful, rubbing, and squeezing them. This immediately chang of your foreplay.

This is a good time to start taking your clothes off, or each other's, if you haven't already. You don't need to say anything. Just start taking your shirt off or lifting theirs up, signaling that it's nakey time.

Once you're naked, restrain yourself.

The natural inclination is to get too excited and go for your partner's genitals as fast as possible. Resist this temptation.

Remember, you're constantly building up tension and releasing it every once in a while.

Instead of going for them as fast as possible, lightly caress your partner around their genitals like you were doing before. Focus on the area around their hips, lower belly, and inner thighs.

You don't have to caress their whole body, but make sure to tease them again. They will be *dying* for you to finally touch them and release them of this amazing desire.

When you're ready, go ahead and lightly touch, rub, and massage their genitals.

How to Stimulate Your Partner's Breasts

If your partner has breasts, squeeze, pull, and massage them gently, but only to a certain extent. You're not trying to tune into Tokyo.

Breasts can be more or less sensitive depending on the individual, and you will be able to tell by how your partner reacts when you stimulate them.

You can also stimulate your partner's nipples, which can produce pleasure signals when touched, rubbed, pulled gently, or sucked on. Try nibbling on them like you would your partner's lips or earlobe.

The Mental Pleasure of Stimulating Your Partner's Butt

When stimulating your partner's butt, there is less biological pleasure involved, but there can be a lot of mental pleasure.

Squeezing it, digging your nails into it, and giving it a good slap gives your foreplay (and your sex) an animalistic dynamic. It's hot. It's raunchy. And it can momentarily wake someone out of a sexual trance and bring them back into the pleasure of the moment.

How to Manually Stimulate the Penis

If your partner has a penis, start working your hands up and down the shaft, touching the head every once in a while. The head is sensitive, and if there isn't any lube or saliva to lessen the friction, it can be quite painful if it's overly stimulated. So be gentle at first.

Also, make your way down to the testicles, gently fondling them, and even further down to the area of skin between the testicles and anus, called the ***perineum***.

Massaging this area while working the shaft is a double whammy of pleasure, as the perineum is home to nerves that correlate directly with pleasure in the penis.

Teasing Your Partner's Vagina While Providing Pleasure

If your partner has a vagina, resist the temptation to enter with your fingers or aggressively stimulate the clitoris straight away.

Tease your partner first. Make light circles with your fingers around the whole expanse of their vulva.

Move down the inner thigh every once in a while, then back up again. Make them crave your touch.

Caress your fingers down the outer lips, barely tickling their skin. Progressively apply more pressure until the lips open up and you reach the vaginal entrance, **but do not enter yet**.

A lot of nerve endings are located here. Take advantage of them.

Rub up and down the expanse of the vaginal entrance. Make a straight line up to the clitoris (the little ball of pleasure located at the north end of the vulva) and then back down. Continue doing this as their vagina gets more lubricated.

Continue rubbing from the vaginal entrance to the clitoris as their sexual arousal mounts.

By now, you should both be *aching* to move things forward. Go ahead and do it.

Direct Stimulation of Your Partner's Genitals

If your partner has a penis, start rhythmically stimulating the penis by wrapping it with your hand and moving your hand up and down, stimulating the entire shaft.

Don't go too fast. You are not trying to end the show in the second act.

Just keep the motion going and feel if they are getting too close to climax. You will be able to tell whether they are getting too close by slight contractions in their shaft and perineum. Their body may also tense up (especially their legs).

If this happens, slow down or completely stop before continuing. You can also continue stimulating the balls or massaging the perineum.

If your partner has a vagina, go ahead and enter with one finger, whichever one is most comfortable for the angle of your hand. There are a number of things you can do from here to stimulate your partner:

- **Angle your finger up towards the roof of the vagina to stimulate the G-Spot**. The G-Spot is a cluster of nerve endings located on the roof of the vagina about 2 inches in. It's famous for its pleasure potential. A misconception is that it stands apart from other areas of pleasure in the vagina. In fact, it is part of a vast *clitoral network* comprised of multiple parts (*She Comes First,* Ian Kerner). Angle your finger up, applying pressure to the G-Spot as you move your finger in and out.

- **Take your finger out, trail up the vulva to the clitoris and back down again into the vagina**. During foreplay, you want to stimulate the clitoris every once in a while, getting it accustomed to your touch and coaxing the little love button out from under the clitoral hood.

- **Instead of going in and out, keep your finger inside and move it up and down**. Move your whole hand. Don't just wiggle your finger. Focus on applying pressure to the G-Spot every time your hand moves up. The vagina is a strong organ. This is where babies come out of, so you can apply some force. But if it starts to hurt your partner, tone it down.

- **Try different variations and pay attention to how your partner reacts**. This is related to what I mentioned previously, called "sexual intuition," which will be discussed in a later chapter. Basically, whatever sexual move pops into your head, don't be afraid to try it. You may end up finding the perfect way to give your partner an intense amount of pleasure. The key is paying attention to how their body reacts to it. Does their breathing deepen? Do they moan louder? Does their body start shaking involuntarily? Do they tell you to keep going? If so, you've struck gold. If not, or if they seem indifferent to it, switch it up.

You can enter with additional fingers at any time as long as their vaginal muscles have relaxed and gotten accustomed to penetration.

As one of you starts going full force in stimulating the other, the other partner will probably follow suit. But if they don't, and you would like them to, use our suggestion technique and nudge their hand towards your genitals.

You can also tell them verbally, in a sexual way of course. Phrase your request with one of these lines or a similar version:

- I want you to _____. (ex. jack me off, finger me)
- Do _____ to me while I do _____ to you.
- I would love it if you did _____ to me right now.
- I love it when you do _____ to me.

Phrasing it like this helps you avoid asking for it and seeming needy, and it also frames it in a way that will make your partner excited to do it for you.

Try whispering your request in their ear as well. This works especially well if you're the more dominant partner.

(We'll cover making requests and dirty talk in Chapter 9.)

Closing Thoughts on Foreplay

To recap, foreplay is about constantly giving and taking away pleasure. You are slowly building up the sexual tension and releasing it every once in a while.

Tease your partner. Make them crave your touch. Make them crave your body. Try out new moves that pop into your head, and pay attention to how your partner reacts to them. This will tell you whether to continue or to try something else.

The goal with foreplay is to build a solid foundation of arousal.

Think of it as putting in more work earlier on, in order to reap greater rewards later. You will have to exercise restraint. It's easy to give in and go straight for it. But you and your partner won't get as much out of it.

It will be good sex. But it won't be great sex.

So resist the temptation to go straight to intercourse, and take some time to heat up the cauldron of desire for each other.

There is another crucial aspect of great sex that must not be overlooked.

It can be seen as a gift to your partner, through its one-sided nature.

Can you guess what it is?

Chapter 5

ORAL SEX: FELLATIO AND CUNNILINGUS TECHNIQUES

Oral sex!

Or third base, going down, cunnilingus, fellatio, blowjob, head. There are lots of fun names for this one.

Oral sex is commonly deemed a skill. People are either bad at it, good at it, or mediocre/average.

What I try to preach is that yes, someone can actually be good or bad at giving oral sex, but more often than not, it's the ***sexual compatibility*** of the two people that determines the quality of a given session of oral sex.

As we said before, everyone feels pleasure differently. So if something worked for one partner and gave them astronomical amounts of pleasure, the exact same thing may not work for another partner.

If you have tried everything and you just can't seem to pleasure your partner the way you want to, it may be out of your control for the time being.

What it presents is an opportunity to find out from your partner what works for them, and maybe learn a cool new way to pleasure someone.

That being said, there is A LOT you can do to educate yourself on the intricacies of oral sex and improve the odds that you will be compatible with more people.

Let's get to it.

How to Give Magnificent Fellatio

Fellatio is the act of stimulating a penis with your mouth. Sounds simple right? Just put your mouth on there and you're good to go.

Not quite. There are some key "do not's" that many aspiring head doctors (so good they could have their Ph. D.) neglect.

Do not...

• Use your teeth. This should be a given. It hurts (unless your partner is into that, by all means go for it).

• Suck the testicles too hard when stimulating them.

• Overstimulate the head (we'll get more into this in a minute).

The reason behind most of these "do not's" is that they are painful and may only be pleasurable in extenuating circumstances when your partner finds them enjoyable.

So if you like doing any of the above to your partner, find out if they like it first, or you may be in for some abrupt and agonizing reactions.

Throughout this process, don't forget about teasing your partner and building up sexual tension. While you *can* go straight into fellatio, or any oral sex, great sex dictates taking an extra couple minutes to make your partner really crave it.

Practicing Fantastic Fellatio Technique

Before direct stimulation-

Kiss your partner's body repeatedly, slowly moving down to their crotch area.

Get right over their penis, but do not touch it yet. Kiss around their inner thighs, the lower part of their belly, and their hips. Run your fingers in circles around their crotch area.

Before putting your mouth straight on it, give it subtle kisses and licks, teasing your partner and making them practically beg for more.

You will end up giving it to them, just not quite yet (remember – you are having sex with their mind just as much as their body).

When you're ready, and you feel like they can't take it anymore, give in and release them of that sexual tension.

The two types of fellatio-

Fellatio can be broken up into two parts:

1. Dedicated Fellatio — Fellatio as the sexual activity in and of itself

2. Pre-Sex Fellatio — Fellatio as a precursor to more sexual activity (such as foreplay).

1) Dedicated Fellatio — As the sexual activity in and of itself

If it's the sexual activity in and of itself, **pleasure** is the name of the game. Penises respond to rhythmic stimulation:

Once you've found the sweet spot – *keep going*.

Although it's really hot if you can get your mouth as far onto your partner's penis as possible, this isn't always the most pleasurable. By all means, don't shy away from doing it, because it can provide immense cognitive pleasure (it's super hot for your partner).

But when you're trying to bring your partner to climax, the optimal distance is maybe a quarter of an inch from the back of your throat. Of course, this will differ according to their size and individual response to pleasure, but when you start rhythmically stimulating the penis, going in about this distance should be optimal.

Another key is to make sure their penis is well lubricated. In general, the more saliva you can get onto it, the better. This will reduce friction and make your fellatio feel even more amazing.

Try spitting on their penis as well. This can provide cognitive pleasure *and* physical pleasure once you begin stimulating it again.

Remember, the head is very sensitive, but it is also a crucial part of giving your partner an orgasm. When you first start going down on your partner, stimulate the head periodically. Focus on the shaft and fondle their balls with your hand, then come up and focus on the head, then back down again.

As the head gets more lubricated and accustomed to stimulation, you can progressively stimulate it more and more. Once your partner is ready to have an orgasm, stimulating their head gives them the final jolt to get over the sexual precipice to orgasm.

You can also try using your hand in combination with your mouth as your partner nears orgasm. Wrap your hand around their shaft with your thumb and index finger touching your lips. As your head goes down, move your hand with it. As your head comes up, follow it with your hand. This will stimulate the entire penis with that rhythmic motion you're looking for.

2) Pre-Sex Fellatio — As a precursor to sex

I'm classifying the second type of fellatio as "Pre-Sex Fellatio" (or as a part of foreplay).

There is reason why I define this type as separate from the previous one.

Generally, when you're planning to continue sexual activity, it's in yours and your partner's best interests for them to hold off on having an orgasm. If your partner has an orgasm now, you will have to wait for the refractory period to end before you two can continue again.

Again, everyone has a different refractory period (the time between the most recent orgasm and when an individual is physically capable of having another one or continuing stimulation). If this period happens to be very short, by all means, do what works best for your particular situation. But for the general population, my advice is to provide pleasure and stimulation, but hold off on giving them an orgasm.

With this type of fellatio, and with any type of oral sex, enthusiasm is what gives your partner satisfaction and makes oral sex so awesome. The opposite, AKA acting like it's a chore or that it's something that *has* to be done, makes your partner feel like it's not worth it.

So be enthusiastic. This means going as deep as you can, gagging yourself, spitting on it, licking it up and down. Basically, showing that you love what you're doing (even if you actually don't).

Work the balls, massage the perineum (the area of skin below the balls), and if your partner is comfortable with it, massage or lick the anus (be mindful of hygiene concerns, which will be discussed in the chapter on anal sex). The anus contains pleasurable nerve endings just like those in our genitalia.

Be enthusiastic in your approach to fellatio. Give oral sex to their mind just as much as their body. Dig your nails into their legs. Interlock your hands with theirs. Tell them how much you love the way they taste. Tell them what you want them to do you later and what you want to do to them later. Don't be afraid to speak up.

Despite your enthusiasm, keep the ultimate goal of continuing the interaction in the back of your mind. If you feel that your partner is about to have an orgasm, slow down or stop completely. I know it sounds counterintuitive, but if you want to keep the show going, there is no shame in taking five.

The key points to great fellatio:

- No teeth (unless you are both into it).

- Don't suck the testicles too hard or overstimulate the head.

- Resist going for it immediately. Rather, take a couple minutes to build up the sexual tension, until they almost can't take it anymore. Then give it to them.

- Penises respond to rhythmic stimulation.

- If it's the sexual activity in and of itself (Dedicated Fellatio), pleasure is the name of the game.

- Make sure their penis is well lubricated with your saliva.

- Enthusiasm is the crucial element that makes oral sex so awesome.

On to the next one! Who wants to become a cunnilinguist?

The Subtle Art of Cunnilingus

Cunnilingus is the act of stimulating a vagina/vulva with one's tongue and/or mouth.

The framework for this section comes from Ian Kerner's glorious book, *She Comes First: The Thinking Man's Guide to Pleasuring a Woman*. The book is directed at heterosexual men, but he could have easily made it gender and sexual orientation neutral.

He also describes different perspectives on sex that I hadn't been introduced to before. A lot of what he wrote opened my eyes to a more passion-filled side of sexuality.

While much of this information comes from Ian Kerner's book, as always, I will be sprinkling in my own experience as well.

Remember how we broke fellatio up into two types – as the sexual activity in and of itself and as a precursor to sex? When performing cunnilingus, we don't have to do that. The same techniques apply either way because a longer refractory period is less likely to occur.

In fact, with most people that have vaginas, it becomes easier for them to have subsequent orgasms once they have had their first one.

The easiest way to describe cunnilingus is to break it up into phases.

Phase #1 – Teasing and Coaxing

First, tease your partner and coax their genitals into being ready for more consistent stimulation.

As with fellatio, start by kissing down their body towards their crotch area. Inch down slowly, as your partner's mind starts to revel in what's to come.

Kiss in a big circle around their genitals – the lower part of the belly, hips, and inner thighs. Run your fingers along their inner thighs, stopping just before you get to their vulva.

As you continue kissing, make smaller and smaller circles, inching closer to the area they are dying for you to reach. Their cauldron is burning hot now, but they are going to have to wait a little longer for relief.

As you get close to the outer lips, place yourself in a comfortable position that you can sustain. Try lying on your stomach with your head in between your partner's thighs. To reduce strain on your neck, place a pillow under their butt to lift up their pelvis. You can also ask your partner to move to the edge of the bed while you kneel on the floor.

Another cool trick is to periodically rest your head on one of their thighs as you lick them. This provides rest/recovery for you (if you need it) and a different angle for them.

Direct Stimulation-

When you are ready to directly stimulate their vulva (outer lips, inner lips, clitoris, vaginal entrance), start by kissing around the outer lips. Make your partner crave your tongue even more by holding off slightly longer.

At this point, it's a good idea to add some extra moisture to the area. Let saliva fall from your mouth to the top of their vulva. Let it slowly trail down towards the vaginal entrance. Often, your partner won't know it's coming, and will gasp with the sudden feeling of cold wet liquid. This is a good thing.

As your partner should be warmed up now, it's time for the first lick.

Start at the very bottom of their vulva, and lightly graze its expanse all the way up just before touching the clitoris, but do not make contact. You're saving that for later.

Do this about five more times, pausing for a few seconds between each lick. This is the epitome of building up the sexual tension we've been harping on.

When you're ready, use your tongue to part their outer lips and expose the inner labia. There is a high density of nerve endings in this area, but you don't want to stimulate them just yet. Lick between the inner and outer lips, continuing to tease and coax.

You can stop every once in a while, kiss around their vulva again, let saliva fall from your mouth onto their vulva, and resume licking between the inner and outer lips.

After a short while, you should both be ready for phase two.

Phase #2 – The Buildup

This is when stimulation becomes more consistent. You are going to build up the tension so much that it will only take a bit of persistent effort to release it.

You have been licking between the inner and outer lips, with the vaginal entrance exposed. There is an area of tissue *just* above the vaginal entrance and below the clitoris. This area is pleasure-packed with nerve endings, and often one of the best places to focus on when bringing your partner to orgasm. However, we've jumped the gun a little bit, so hold that thought for a moment.

Start from the bottom of the vaginal entrance, just above the perineum. Lick all the way up to the area just below the clitoris, gliding over the sensitive area above the vaginal entrance. Stop here. Do not make contact with the clitoris just yet. Repeat this five times or so.

After one round, lick all the way up, but this time **make contact** with the clitoris and hold the tip of your tongue there for a moment. Your partner has been waiting for this, and may shudder with pleasure at the sudden contact. This is also a good thing.

Repeat this cycle as many times as you like for 10 minutes or so. You want to get the most sensitive areas of your partner's vulva accustomed to consistent stimulation.

You're also coaxing the clitoris, the epicenter of pleasure, out from hiding under the clitoral hood.

Direct stimulation of the clitoris-

Once their clitoris becomes accustomed to the touch of your tongue, you can start applying more direct stimulation.

Start with sideways licks horizontally across the clitoris. Go about a quarter of an inch to each side, grazing the clitoris as your tongue passes over. At this point, it's important to pay attention to how your partner reacts to the pressure you apply.

Possible signs that you should release the pressure:

- Your partner gasps abruptly and holds their breath.
- Your partner digs their nails into your hands, arms, or bed sheets.
- Your partner tells you that it's too much.

Of course, these are only guidelines. Sometimes these reactions mean you're doing the right thing. Only by experimenting will you truly know.

Try lessening your pressure, notice how they react, then judge whether you should apply more or less pressure. Everyone feels pleasure differently. It's your mission to find out how your partner feels it best.

After doing sideways licks for a few minutes, switch to vertical licks up and down the clitoris. Extend your licks all the up to the clitoral shaft (the area just above the clitoris) and back down to the sensitive area of tissue below the clitoris.

You don't need to go too fast. One side-effect of watching porn is thinking that you need to keep your face an inch and a half away from the vulva and lick as fast as possible. This is for the camera man to get a good angle. It is NOT optimized for pleasure and should not be modeled off of (I know this because I made this mistake, among others that I "learned" from porn).

It's actually best to make as much contact as possible with your lips and tongue. Use your saliva as constant moisture, and place your lips over the vulva as you lick, pursing them like you've just bitten into a piece of fruit. This provides extra stimulation for your partner, and takes excess strain off your face and neck muscles.

As you are stimulating the clitoris with your lips around it, trying sucking the clitoris and the surrounding area into your mouth and continue licking. Don't worry, it may be sensitive, but it is a strong organ.

The hard feeling of your teeth and sucking pressure on the area around her clitoris provides a lot of pleasure. Combined with horizontal and vertical licks, and moisture from your saliva, you may have just hit the cunnilingus jackpot.

Whenever you feel like the clitoris is starting to become overly stimulated, revert back to repeatedly licking the entire vulva from bottom to top.

You can also try massaging the perineum (the area of skin between the vulva and anus) any time during cunnilingus. Massaging or licking the anus can also give their clitoris a pleasurable break (as long as your partner is comfortable with it).

Finger stimulation-

Another tip is to insert one or two fingers into the vagina as you lick their clitoris. For some, this feels great and enhances the pleasure. For others, it either doesn't provide any added pleasure or actually lessens it.

Go ahead and try it and see how your partner reacts. Afterwards, ask them if they liked it and if they want you to do it in the future.

Don't just insert your fingers any old way and leave them there. Insert them with a purpose. You can angle them up to the G-Spot (2 inches inside, on the roof of the vagina). You can also insert your fingers and spread them apart, simulating the feeling of being full your partner gets from penetration.

You can also go in and out, stimulating the entrance and inner part of the vagina as you lick the area around their clitoris. Inserting your thumb may also work to provide your partner the feeling of being full if angling two fingers is too much for them or uncomfortable for you. This is a great opportunity to massage the perineum (area below the vulva) as well.

At this point, the sexual tension should be building up immensely. Some partners will remain in this phase for some time before being ready to continue on to the final phase, and that's fine.

The time it takes to reach orgasm differs for everyone and under different circumstances, so be supportive, be patient, and do your best to pleasure them (as they should do for you).

Phase #3 – The Release

It's time for the grand finale. Let's release your partner of the tension you've built up over the past two phases.

The clitoris is going to be the main focus of your attention, but you can also expand your reach to the clitoral network as a whole, which you will see soon enough.

Start this phase with consistent licks over the clitoris, switching between horizontal and vertical every so often. When licking horizontal, go about a quarter of an inch to each side. When licking vertical, go up to the clitoral shaft and down to the soft tissue below the clitoris. Keep your lips pursed around the area of the clitoris, sucking in every once in a while.

That is your main focus right there. The clitoris is the ultimate vehicle to get your partner over the pleasure hill to orgasmic release. However, the only reason this is possible is because you spent that time building up sexual tension and arousal. (That's why it isn't wise to skip everything you just did and head straight here, however tempting it may be.)

By now, hopefully you have gained a feel for how sensitive your partner's clitoris is and how much stimulation it can handle. If their clitoris is too sensitive for constant stimulation, focus your licks on the sensitive tissue a few centimeters below the clitoris, making contact with the clitoris every so often.

Sometimes, even if your partner's clitoris isn't too sensitive, this is still the area you want to focus on, so give it a try either way and see how your partner reacts.

As your partner gets closer and closer to orgasm, you simply have to find the final licking sequence to get them there. From here, you have two options, and they will seem contradictory but both work to get the same result.

1. Increase the speed and intensity of your licks, focusing all of your pressure on either the clitoris or the area below the clitoris.
2. Decrease the speed entirely. Keep licking lightly, and perform a forceful lick every 10-15 seconds.

I know. Sounds like I'm bullshitting right? I'm not.

Depending on your partner, their sweet spot may fall somewhere near these two extremes.

The good news is: All you have to do is try out both extremes and see which one works best. Then you have found your moneymaker.

Once you've found it, keep going and don't let up. Your tongue may be tired. Your face muscles may be cramping. But don't stop – for the sake of your partner's pleasure. Keep going until you feel their body reach orgasmic release.

Utilizing the clitoral network-

You just brought your partner to orgasm simply through one part of the clitoral network: The clitoris. Now let's see how you can incorporate other parts of it.

As you are following the above steps, insert one or two fingers into their vagina and stimulate the G-Spot as well. Either massage it while keeping your fingers inside, or move them in and out, putting pressure on the G-Spot whenever your fingers are inserted far enough.

While keeping your fingers of one hand in, you can also reach around and place your other hand on top of their belly and pelvic area, just above where the G-Spot rests. Apply pressure to this area. This will further stimulate that cluster of nerve endings.

Again with the fingers, you can try inserting them inside in the shape of a "peace sign" and angling them downwards. There are two parts of the clitoral network that run down the sides of the vagina from the clitoris itself, called the *clitoral crura*. By angling your fingers this way, you will stimulate this area in addition to licking the clitoris, satisfying a larger portion of the clitoral network.

Concluding Cunnilingus and Oral Sex

Cunnilingus is about coaxing your partner through their sexual response cycle (Excitement, Plateau, Orgasm, and Resolution).

With cunnilingus (and any aspect of sex), the best way to find out what worked and what didn't is to ask your partner afterwards. You'll know whether you stimulated the clitoris too much, whether putting your fingers inside felt amazing or not, what you could have done to make them orgasm harder, etc.

And even if you don't have one or the other of the above body parts, understanding how to pleasure *yourself* is the best way to help your partner pleasure you. If you skipped over either of the above sections for this reason, I urge you to go back and read them. You may discover a way to pleasure yourself you never knew before, and a way to help your partner take you to the highest heights of pleasure.

Who would want to miss out on *that*?

Not me. And I know lots of people who wouldn't want to miss out on the next chapter, either.

Chapter 6

ANAL SEX

I wouldn't be surprised if many readers have skipped everything above and headed straight here.

(You naughty dog, you.)

Anal sex is a hot topic, and rightly so. We're only just beginning to enter an era where this aspect of sex is becoming commonplace for everyone, no matter their sexual orientation.

However, this means there is still a lot of misinformation and misconception out there, which I will try to clear up as much as possible in this chapter.

I'm going to break this up by discussing the science and biology behind anal sex first. Then I'll get into some best practices.

I know Wikipedia isn't exactly a credible source, but I have done my research and haven't found anything more comprehensive than their page. I compiled most of the following biological information using Wikipedia as a guide, and have not included anything that I haven't read elsewhere before.

Why Anal Sex Can Be Pleasurable – The Biology of Our Butts

The keyword here is "can." The fact of the matter is, it's pleasurable for some people and for others it just hurts.

But there are biological and mental reasons why it's pleasurable for many people, and there are things you can do to make anal play more pleasurable (I'll be using "anal play" as a general term that encompasses all sexual activity involving the anus).

First off, the outer part of the anus (the visible area), two sphincter muscles, and the rectum, are all made of soft tissue that's filled with pleasure-inducing nerve endings, just like the ones in other sexual organs.

Two muscles control the opening and closing of the anus: The external sphincter and the internal sphincter. Exercising control over these two muscles is a big determinant in whether any type of anal play, whether it be intercourse, toys, fingering, etc., is pleasurable or not.

The outer two thirds of the anus can be sensitive to stimulation, and as you go further in, it becomes less sensitive to gentle touch, but more responsive to pressure.

For those with penises, the main biological reason why anal play can be pleasurable involves the prostate. Anal stimulation of the prostate can be very pleasurable, because it's similar to the nerve ending cluster of the G-Spot.

Stimulation of this area can produce more intense orgasms than penile stimulation, causing involuntary body movements like the ones that can be produced from G-Spot orgasms. It can also produce deeper, longer lasting orgasms than penile stimulation alone. In order to stimulate the prostate, angle the inserted object diagonally towards the belly button.

For those with vaginas, several biological reasons exist as to why anal play can be pleasurable. First, anal stimulation is said to be connected to stimulation of the clitoral network. Remember the vaginal crura? If not, they are the two parts of the clitoral network that run down the inner part of the vagina, stemming from the clitoris itself (we used the "peace sign" technique to stimulate these during cunnilingus). These can be indirectly stimulated through anal play.

The G-Spot can also be stimulated through anal sex, as the vaginal and rectal cavities are quite close to each other. Angled correctly in certain instances, anal stimulation this way can produce G-Spot orgasms. Manually stimulating the G-Spot, clitoris, and vulva while having anal sex can also make anal play more pleasurable.

In all body types, anal play can produce enjoyable sensations through stimulation of the *pudendal nerve*. This nerve indirectly connects to the *perineal nerve*, which is located in the perineum and connects to either the *dorsal nerve of the penis* or the *dorsal nerve of the clitoris*, indirectly stimulating **both types of genitals.**

Best Practices for Safe Anal Play

This must be stated first: For those partaking in penis-to-anus anal sex, unprotected anal sex in this way leaves both partners more vulnerable to STIs than any other type of sex. Why? There are several reasons:

- The tissues in the anus and rectum are relatively thin and the anus doesn't produce its own lubrication. This causes tissue breakage to happen more often. This breakage provides a pathway for harmful bacteria and viruses to pass through and enter the bloodstream. Toys are not invincible. They can carry bacteria and viruses on them, as well, if not cleaned properly.

- Condoms are more likely to break during anal sex due to the nature of the rectum.

- The anus is predominantly meant to carry and expel feces, which contains a host of harmful bacteria that becomes more easily transmitted during unprotected anal sex.

The above bullet points are all reasons why safe sex should be practiced by everyone who engages in anal play, not only by penis-to-anus practitioners. Here are some tips for safer anal play, courtesy of Wikipedia and WebMD:

- No matter what object is being inserted, whether it's a penis, finger, dildo, vibrator, strap-on dildo, etc, always use a condom. Yes, I realize just as much as anyone that condoms aren't as fun. But what's worse – having a little less feeling due to a condom, or getting a life changing STI such as HIV? It's your life. You have to live with the decisions you make.

- If you or your partner have been diagnosed with an STI, avoid anal play until the ailment has been treated and cured.

- Clean the area thoroughly and empty the bowels before engaging in anal play.

- Clean any object that was used during anal play, ESPECIALLY before using it for any other sexual activity. For toys, they usually come with specific cleaning

- instructions. Cleaning products are also available for purchase. Follow those instructions and use those products.

- When engaging in anilingus (licking the outer part of the anus) the use of a dental dam or plastic wrap is recommended.

- See a doctor ASAP if you notice bleeding, sores, or discharge after anal play.

My Suggestions for Enjoying Anal Play

- Use a fair amount of lubrication, and a condom, to make entry of the object smoother and less painful.

- If you are the receiving partner, focus on relaxing your sphincter muscles as the object is inserted. Most of the pain is caused when people react by squeezing their butt muscles. This is the opposite of what you want to do.

- Again, if you are the receiving partner, try pushing out a bit with your abdominal muscles as the object is being inserted. This should help your sphincter muscles relax. Also, try laying on your stomach or side rather than your back.

- If you are the partner inserting the object, make sure you're using enough lubrication. Go slowly and listen to your partner as the object is inserted. If they tell you to stop, then stop. If they tell you to take it out, take it out. If they say you can put it in further, then you may do so. Obey their wishes. It's their body.

Closing Anal Sex

Anal is yet another infrequently traversed sexual territory that is thrilling to pursue for many people. It's exciting to try something new, especially if it can be pleasurable as well (and in some cases, VERY pleasurable).

But, especially with anal play, it's important to keep safety in mind. No amount of pleasure is worth the stress, anxiety, physical ailment, and cost of getting an STI or other infection. It's also not worth the guilt of transmitting one, so get tested regularly and know the status of your body.

The precautionary measures I outlined are not meant to deter you from anal sex. They're meant to keep you safe as you navigate it.

The topic of the next chapter is one of the most talked about aspects of sex.

If you google "sex positions," it returns 2.9 million results. People obviously care about how they contort themselves in the sack.

But out of 2.9 million results, how do you pick the best of the best for your own sex life?

I believe I have stumbled on a few you will find worth considering.

Chapter 7

16 POWERFUL POSITIONS FOR THE HOTTEST SEX AND DEEPEST INTIMACY

When you search for sex positions on the internet, you will find that most sources list the same positions over and over again. While this isn't necessarily a bad thing, they typically don't tell you why they chose them.

For our purposes, I'm only going to include the best of the best that I've found. These are the positions that provide the most pleasure, the hottest sex, the deepest intimacy, and give you the best opportunities to multitask (which will be discussed in a later chapter).

I have broken them up into penetrative, non-penetrative, and oral sex positions. Penetrative includes any object, such as a penis, toy, or strap-on dildo, being used to enter your partner. Non-penetrative includes the rubbing together of genitals and mutual masturbation.

I'll be describing the positions in terms of how both partners should be situated and what benefits each position offers.

Good sex requires different positions. Great sex requires POWERFUL positions.

Let's break 'em down.

Powerful Penetrative Positions

#1 *Missionary With Legs in the Air*

Description-

- The penetrating partner is on top and the receiving partner is on bottom.

- Instead of regular missionary with the receiving partner's legs spread out on the bed, the receiving partner spreads their legs about two feet apart and lifts them up in the air towards the ceiling, keeping them in front of their partner. Their body becomes an L shape.

- The receiving partner rests the back of their legs against the chest and shoulders of their partner, typically with their knees bending over their partner's shoulders and their hamstrings on their partner's chest.

- The penetrating partner leans forward, with their head between their partner's legs, and put their hands on the bed next to their partner's head, with their arms straight. This should angle their partner's pelvis upwards.

- Finally, the penetrating partner enters.

Benefits-

- Great angle for stimulating the G-Spot, anus, and/or prostate.

- The pressure of the receiving partner's legs provides some relief for the penetrating partner's arms.

- The receiving partner is somewhat constrained, which can be a turn on for many people.

Variation-

- Instead of two legs towards the ceiling, the receiving partner only puts one of their legs up, providing a different angle of stimulation.

#2 Missionary While Grabbing the Butt

Description-

- Regular missionary position with the penetrating partner on top and receiving partner on bottom, except the penetrating partner lies completely on top, resting their weight on their partner.

- With their head to the side of their partner's head, possibly resting on the pillow, the penetrating partner reaches down with both hands and grabs hold of their partner's butt.

Benefits-

- Allows the penetrating partner to pull their partner in towards them and thrust at the same time.

- Creates more bodily contact, increasing intimacy.

- Better angle than regular missionary for stimulating the G-Spot, anus, and/or prostate.

#3 Receiving Partner Lying Sideways and Penetrating Partner On Top

Description-

- The receiving partner lies on their side with legs bent at a 90 degree angle.
- The penetrating partner enters from the top, so the front of penetrating partner is facing the side of the receiving partner.
- The penetrating partner kneels within the 90 degree angle of their partner's legs, positioning their pelvis to enter their partner.
- The penetrating partner leans forward and places their hands, arms, or elbows on both sides of their partner to hold themselves up.

Benefits-

- Different angle of stimulation.
- Can still kiss each other, heightening intimacy.

Variation-

- The penetrating partner grabs their partner's top leg and puts it over the corresponding arm.
- This widens either the vagina or anus for easier entry, and creates a different dynamic of constraint.

#4 Legs in the Air on the Edge of the Bed

Description-

- Similar to #1. The receiving partner lies on their back, puts their legs together and raises them up to the ceiling so their body is in an L shape. Except this time, they are on the edge of the bed with the penetrating partner standing up.

- The penetrating partner wraps or holds on to their partner's legs for thrusting leverage, and may have to bend their knees down a bit to enter their partner. However, this partner does not lean over yet, like in #1, but stays standing straight.

Benefits-

- The penetrating partner gets great leverage by holding onto or wrapping around their partner's legs.

- Another optimal angle for stimulating the G-Spot, anus, and/or prostate.

Variation-

- Can have legs spread open rather than together.

- Can do the same as #1, with legs spread, hamstrings against the chest, and penetrating partner leaning over their partner while holding themselves up.

#5 Doggy Style With Receiving Partner Curling Towards Other Partner

Description-

- Receiving partner goes on their hands and knees while the penetrating partner gets on their knees and enters from behind.

- Instead of being on their hands, the receiving partner then rests one shoulder on the bed and angles their head to the opposite side, angling their back downwards towards the bed. The receiving partner should be able to look back and see their partner.

- The receiving partner rests their arms on the bed towards their partner.

- The penetrating partner holds on to their partner's hips for thrusting leverage.

Benefits-

- Better angle for deeper penetration.

- Increased arousal by both partners being able to lock eyes with one another, and especially for the receiving partner who gets to see their partner entering them from behind.

- Penetrating partner can get good leverage by holding onto their partner's hips and waist.

Variation-

- The receiving partner bends their knees further and lowers their pelvis down closer to the bed. They then reach back with their hands and wrap their arms around their legs, curling themselves further into a ball.

#6 Doggy Style With Penetrating Partner Squatting Over

Description-

- The receiving partner is on their hands and knees in doggy style position.

- Instead of being on their knees as well, the penetrating partner stands with their feet on either side of their partner, squatting down until they are at the right height to enter. The receiving partner may need to angle their pelvis upwards to help with entry.

- If the penetrating partner is comfortable, they can thrust like this. Otherwise, if they need more balance they can place their hands on the back, shoulders, or hips of their partner while squatting.

Benefits-

- Allows for deeper penetration.

- This angle from behind is better for hitting the G-Spot, anus, and/or prostate.

- The penetrating partner can use gravity to help them thrust.

Variation-

- Similar to the previous position (#5 - Doggy Style With Receiving Partner Curling Towards Other Partner), the receiving partner can angle their back down towards the bed, reach their arms back towards their partner, and curl themselves into a ball. This allows for further comfort during deep penetration and a different angle of stimulation. It also increases intimacy by being able to see each other's faces.

#7 From Behind With Receiving Partner Laying On Stomach

Description-

- The receiving partner lies flat on their stomach with their legs out straight and close together.
- The penetrating partner straddles their partner, with their knees on either side, leans forward, and uses their hands and arms to hold them up while entering their partner.

Benefits-

- Makes the vagina/anus tighten for increased pleasure of both partners.
- A comfortable position for both partners.
- Allows for a lot of multitasking, including hair pulling, kissing and sucking the neck/back, and manual stimulation (hand) of the genitals of the receiving partner.

Variation-

- The penetrating partner lies fully on the receiving partner, without holding themselves up, increasing bodily contact and intimacy.
- The penetrating partner can also reach under and provide manual stimulation to their partner's genitals.
- Provides opportunity to kiss from behind.

#8 Lying Down Sideways Penetration From Behind

Description-

- The receiving partner lies on their side with knees bent at around and 90 degree angle.

- The penetrating partner lies on their side behind them, entering as they would in regular doggy style and using their partner's hip(s) as leverage.

Benefits-

- Hugely intimate position, as it resembles cuddling.

- Provides a lot of opportunity for multitasking, including hair pulling, kissing from behind, manual simulation of the genitals, and constraint by pulling back and locking the receiving partner's arms.

Variation-

- The penetrating partner lifts up the top leg of the receiving partner, either holding it up or placing it on top of their own. This expands the vagina/anus allowing for more comfortable penetration.

#9 Receiving Partner On Top (with variations)

Description-

- The penetrating partner lies on their back with the receiving partner straddling them.

- The receiving partner sits on their partner as they enter them.

- The receiving partner moves their body in a way that stimulates both partners.

Benefits-

- The receiving partner gets to control rhythm and stimulation.

- The receiving partner gains the more dominant role and can exercise more control.

- The penetrating partner becomes the more submissive role.

- The receiving partner is able to move in a way that best stimulates them, and can control depth of penetration.

- Provides opportunity for either partner to manually stimulate the receiving partner's genitals in addition to penetration.

Variations-

- Instead of straddling their partner on their knees, the receiving partner squats over, bending their knees far enough to have their partner enter them. They can place their hands on their partner's shoulders, chest, stomach, or the pillow/bed for added stability and control.

- The receiving partner sits with full penetration and rolls their hips back and forth as they straddle their partner.

- The receiving partner moves up and down, similar to the thrusting action of the penetrating partner.

- The receiving partner lies forward with their weight on the penetrating partner, and rolls their body back and forth or moves up and down. The penetrating partner (on bottom) can also place their hands on their partner's hips or butt to control the rhythm.

- The receiving partner arches backward, instead of forward, and reaches backward placing their hands on either their partner's legs or the bed for balance. The receiving partner then moves in a way that is great for stimulating the G-Spot, anus, and/or prostate.

- The receiving partner faces the opposite direction while straddling their partner, with their butt facing their partner. The receiving partner can put their hands on either the bed or their partner's legs for added balance and control.

- The receiving partner faces the opposite direction, like before, but on their hands and feet facing the ceiling (so their back is towards their partner and they are in a "spider crawl" position). They then lower their hips down enough for their partner to enter. The penetrating partner relieves some of their partner's muscular strain by supporting their hips or lower back with their hands. The penetrating partner then uses that leverage to thrust.

Powerful Non-Penetrative Positions (Wikipedia)

#1 Rubbing Together of the Genitals

Description/Variations-

- One partner positions themselves in between their partner's thighs and rubs their genitals or a similar object (such as a strap-on dildo) on their partner's genitals.

- In the case of two people with vaginas, both people face each other positioning their legs to make contact with each other's vulva in order to rub them together. Sometimes called *scissoring*.

- In the case of two people with penises, both people position themselves in order to rub their penises together. Sometimes called *frot or frottage*.

Benefits-

- Risk of unwanted pregnancy dramatically decreases.

- Provides pleasure and intimacy for those who are uncomfortable with penetrative sexual activity.

#2 *Mutual Masturbation*

Description-

- Both partners lie next to each other in a way that provides easy manual stimulation of each other's genitals.

- Can lie on their backs, on their sides facing each other, both partners facing the same way, or with one partner on their back and the other on their side facing their partner.

Benefits-

- Risk of unwanted pregnancy dramatically decreases.

- Provides pleasure and intimacy for those who are uncomfortable with penetrative sexual activity.

Powerful Oral Sex Positions

#1 68-ing (variation of 69)

Description-

- Similar to the popular "69" position, where one partner lies on their back and the other straddles their genitals over their partner's face, facing the opposite direction and allowing oral access to both partner's genitals (can also be done side-by-side).

- One partner provides oral stimulation to the partner that is lying down, while they orient their body to give their partner manual access to stimulate their genitals.

Benefits-

- Good for foreplay and warming up both partners.

#2 Fellatio Variations

Description-

- The giving partner (the one performing the oral sex) lies on their back with their head hanging off the bed. The receiving partner (the one receiving the oral sex) enters their mouth while standing off the bed, allowing for thrusting. Receiving partner can also reach over and stimulate their partner's genitals at the same time. Can also be done with the giving partner lying on their stomach.

- The receiving partner (receiving oral sex) lies on their back with their legs hanging off the edge of the bed. The giving partner kneels off the bed and provides oral.

#3 Cunnilingus Variations

Description-

- The receiving partner lies on their back with a pillow (or multiple) under their butt in order to lift up their pelvis. The giving partner positions their head in between the thighs of the receiving partner.

- The receiving partner lies on their back with their legs hanging off the edge of the bed. The giving partner kneels off the bed and provides oral. The giving partner can also place the receiving partner's legs over their own shoulders.

Michael's Powerful Position

#1 Gravity

Description-

- I have never seen this position anywhere else, so as far as I'm concerned, I invented it. It's a penetrative position.

- The receiving partner is off the bed and places their shoulder blades on the ground (they are going to be practically upside down) with their back resting against the side of the bed. You may want to place a pillow underneath their head and shoulder blades.

- The receiving partner's legs are spread apart and in the air reaching towards the ceiling.

- The penetrating partner extends their legs on the bed, with their upper body hanging off the bed being supported in a horizontal manner by their hands and arms. They are now in position to enter.

- The penetrating partner uses gravity to thrust every time they move their hips up towards the ceiling and back down.

Benefits-

- It's awesome.

Note that any of these positions can be adapted to use sex toys as well. And when attempting a new position, make sure you're taking the necessary safety precautions not to injure yourself or your partner. Some positions are acrobatic endeavors.

When you first start learning new positions, I suggest taking them one by one instead of trying to go through all of them in a single session. It can be a little stressful trying to remember ten new positions you learned that day. Focus on one at a time and you will memorize each as they become a part of your sexual arsenal.

And don't forget to have fun. Trying new positions is a great activity to share with your partner or partners. Talk about them, play around with what works and what doesn't, and find the top rotation of positions you can stick to that provide the most fun and pleasure.

(In the chapter on transitioning, we will break down these positions further. You will also learn a simple way to remember them and incorporate them into your sex life. So don't worry if this chapter was a little overwhelming.)

Can you guess what's next?

Toys!

And no, not the Legos you used to play with. Although, I'm sure you could make something useful out of them for the bedroom.

Chapter 8

HOW SEX TOYS CAN IMPROVE YOUR SEX LIFE

The first sex toy I ever used was a dildo. After that, a trip to the sex shop for Valentine's Day started a couple month long foray into the incorporation of toys into my sex life. It's one of the best decisions I ever made.

They are not only a quick and efficient way to take your sex life to the next level, but they're super fun to mess around with. They can do things we simply can't do, or at least not as skillfully (like vibrate).

However, it's important not to think of them as *replacements*, but rather *enhancements* of you, your partner(s), and the sex life you already have together.

The name of the game is pleasure, connection, fun, and intimacy. Sex toys help with all of that. By themselves, they can only accomplish a mere fraction of it.

So for people who are hesitant to venture into the world of these devices because of an insecurity you have about them (like I had), trust me when I say it's completely unfounded and you are truly missing out on an exciting aspect of sexuality, not to mention you may be leaving your partner hanging.

There are a number of directions I could have gone with this chapter, but I decided to focus it purely on using sex toys while having sex itself. I also decided to focus on how to use them to optimize the pleasure of both partners.

There are TONS to choose from. It can be quite daunting the moment you step into the sex shop or the online store loads on your computer screen.

Dildos, vibrators, BDSM devices, masturbators, anal stimulators, dolls, edible underpants – the list goes on and on. And within each type of toy are different sub-categories meant for different pleasure goals. So how am I going to narrow this down?

I'm only going to go over the main ones. Why? Because once you understand how they work and have experienced them, that's when you gain a strong enough background knowledge to choose the ones that are REALLY going to enhance your experience.

You will also feel much more comfortable starting out with these than some of the more intricate ones. I've also included links to examples of each to give you a better idea of what I'm talking about.

Diddling Around with Dildos

Dildos are typically made out of a silicone, silicone-type material, or glass and have a phallic shape (the general shape of a penis).

It's a good beginner's toy because it's not complicated to figure out how to use it. If you have a penis, you already know how. Use it like you would your penis.

The following suggestions can be practiced as a part of foreplay, as a break from intercourse in the middle of a session, or whenever it tickles your fancy.

- If you're using a dildo on your partner and they haven't been penetrated yet, enter them slowly and be attentive to how they react. Using a good amount of lube is also recommended.

- Angle the toy towards the G-Spot and/or prostate for maximum pleasure. It can also be used to stimulate the clitoris and/or outer part of the anus or perineum as well.

- In the case of penetrative sex for those who have a vagina, dildos can be used for double penetration (stimulating the vagina with the penis, and the anus with the dildo) or the other way around.

- Strap-on dildos also fall under this category and can be used in any of the above ways.

- You can also find double-penetration dildos, which can be used to stimulate one partner or to be shared between two partners (be aware of hygiene concerns).

- Dildos can also have a vibrating component. The most common are "rabbit" vibrating dildos which have a protrusion from one side, meant to stimulate either the clitoris or the anus.

- There are also dildos meant for anal stimulation. The most common are referred to as "butt plugs," and have a splayed bottom so the toy doesn't get lodged inside the rectum.

Example dildos to check out:

- Glass Dildo with Ribbed Sides
- "Rabbit" Dildo with Vibration

Vibrators – Bite-sized Pleasure That Packs a Punch

Vibrators are usually made of plastic and generally come in smaller sizes. But these little Energizer Bunny sex toys pack a powerful punch.

For many, and those who have vaginas especially, the use of a vibrator is one of the only ways they can orgasm during intercourse. For some, this includes masturbation as well.

Either way, using vibrators is one of the best ways to enhance your sex.

- A torpedo vibrator comes in the shape of a miniature torpedo. They're about 2-4 inches in length and are one of the most common vibrators.

- Typically, vibrators have a different settings that allow you to adjust the speed and intensity of the vibration.

- For those who have a vagina, focus most of your efforts on and around the clitoris. Pay attention to how your partner is reacting. When using a vibrator, the clitoris can become overstimulated rather quickly. Stimulation above, to the side, and on the sensitive tissue below the clitoris might be more pleasurable for your partner.

- For those with a penis, using a vibrator on the head and/or testicles can be pleasurable as well.

- For anal play, focus vibration where the highest density of nerve endings are – the outer tissue, inner two-thirds, and the prostate or area close to the G-Spot.

- Vibrators truly stand out during sexual intercourse. As long as you are in a position where either you or your partner can reach a hand to a part of the other partner's genitals, vibrators can be used. For G-Spot or prostate stimulation, I have found that the best position is either missionary or the first position we described, "Missionary With Legs in the Air." During these positions, penetration is providing intense stimulation on the inner part of the genitals, so you can intensify the experience by using a vibrator to stimulate the outer part of the genitals.

Example vibrators to check out:

- Typical Torpedo Vibrator
- A Popular Type of Massage Vibrator
- Dual-Stimulation Vibrator

Vibrating Rings

Commonly called "penis rings," vibrating rings are just as their name describes – rings that vibrate. Don't worry, they're elastic and usually the part that vibrates is protruding outward.

- For penetrative sex, wearing the ring over the object that is penetrating can add pleasure for both partners.

- For the receiving partner, make sure the ring is positioned so it can make contact with your genitals as your partner thrusts. It should also make the entire penetrating object vibrate as well.

- As the penetrating partner, it's your job to control the stimulation. Rather than constant continuous thrusting, try slow and careful movements. Pause when you are all the way in and the ring has made contact with your partner. Allow the feeling to soak in. Then pull out suddenly, and move in extremely slowly again, teasing your partner. They'll be dying for you to go all the way in. Make them crave it before giving it to them. Don't forget our old motto of give and take.

- You can also find tongue vibrating rings which are meant for cunnilingus. In my experience, they flat out suck, so I wouldn't spend too much money if you plan on buying one. It's an awesome concept, but the execution is awful. Using it is almost like performing cunnilingus while your tongue is numb, because you can't feel what you're touching. I wouldn't recommend it, but hey, maybe you will be more skilled than me.

Example vibrating rings to check out:

- Trojan Brand Vibrating Ring
- Vibrating Tongue Ring

Kinky and Restrictive Devices

Constraint is a turn on for many people. It helps define and play out the sexual roles of domination and submission. However, a common complaint is one partner wanting to kink up their sex life while the other doesn't feel comfortable with it.

There are numerous psychological reasons behind this. But the bottom line is that you two should progress slowly, carefully, and supportively. Both partners need to have a high level of trust and must know when to stop before things go too far.

That being said, there are some fun introductory items to use that aren't too crazy and will still add an entirely new dynamic to your sex life.

- **Blindfolds**. Putting a blindfold on one partner can be extremely sexy. The partner that's blindfolded is suddenly engorged in a world of mystery, while the other is given the perfect opportunity to be creative. Their partner won't know what's about to happen to them until it happens. The partner without the blindfold should take this opportunity to tease them like crazy. Run your fingers up their body. Barely graze over their private parts. Make them crave knowing what's going to happen next. Then make it happen. Again, the level of trust must be high, but this is a great place to start.

- **Rope Ties**. As far as constraint goes, rope ties should be your first stop. You can tie up any appendages and restrict their range of motion. By doing this, you give your partner something to flex against while they're being stimulated, which can help them orgasm. There is also a lot of cognitive pleasure involved, as one partner submits control to the other. It's a fun way to play out certain fantasies. However, proceed with caution. Tying people up certain ways can cause injury.

- **Handcuffs**. These provide similar pleasure to rope ties, but the cognitive pleasure of being handcuffed is different from being tied up. Handcuffs are usually made of metal as well, which can be painful. Try to find a pair that has a cushiony or protective covering.

Example kinky and restrictive devices to check out:

- Padded Leather Blindfold
- Rope Tie and Vibrating Dildo
- Cushioned Handcuffs

Those are the main introductory toys that I decided to include. Of course, there are loads more. A quick Google search is evidence of that.

If you would like to check out more of what's out there, here are a few online stores:

- Adam and Eve
- Spencer's
- Pure Romance
- Amazon – Sex Toys Department

Look at sex toys as a way to introduce a kinkier side to your sex life. Challenge yourself to see just how high you can increase the pleasure of you and your partner. It's an interesting endeavor, and worthwhile once you take the plunge.

This next chapter discusses something that literally changed my sex life in one night.

Enough said.

Chapter 9

GETTING VOCAL IN THE BEDROOM A SIMPLE ACT THAT CAN TAKE YOUR SEX LIFE TO THE NEXT LEVEL

One of my biggest sex life regrets is not becoming vocal in the bedroom sooner. The night I started talking during sex is the night my sex life changed forever.

This stuff is HUGE, and it can make a big improvement in your sex life in a short amount of time.

Talking during sex, or dirty talk, can feel weird for some people. Some people absolutely hate it, and some love it. The people who love it think that sex is lacking without it.

When it comes down to it, it doesn't matter what other people think.

What matters is whether **you** like it and whether **your partner** likes it. You also want to know how to introduce dirty talk to your sex life, because it can feel strange in the beginning. My goal for this section is to help you discover both.

How I Started Talking During Sex

Before that fateful night, I had no desire whatsoever to speak up in the bedroom.

I had no clue what to say. I figured that whatever I said would come out wrong or lame. And I thought that sex talk mostly happened in porn, not in real life.

I wasn't completely silent. I made grunts and moaned if something felt really good. But I definitely wasn't saying the type of stuff I say now, which will be discussed in a minute.

I decided to try dirty talk after reading about it in *The Men's and Women's Health Big Book of Sex*. It discussed how big of a turn on it can be. To be honest, they downplayed the possibilities.

I decided why not? Let's give it a go and see what happens. My first sentence went something like:

"I love your pussy."

Not exactly monumental stuff on paper, but in the heat of the moment it was awesome. My partner loved it and started talking back to me, and the hotness level skyrocketed (we also happened to be having sex between some bushes on our way home from the bars, so that could have helped a bit).

I started saying more after that, talking about how good my partner felt, how I couldn't wait to come inside her, what I wanted to do to her next. It was great, and she complimented me on it afterwards.

Since that night, I talk during sex almost every time I get the chance. Sometimes we're trying to be quiet or we're having a quickie, so there are instances when I make sure to keep my mouth shut. But other than that, I let the vocals flow and I can see the difference it makes compared to being silent.

How Being Vocal Changed My Sex Life, and How it Can Change Yours As Well

First, I immediately noticed how it enhanced the balance of dominance. It's one thing to be on top constraining your partner, and another to do it while whispering in their ear, "I'm going to have my way with you." If you can imagine that, you can imagine how powerful it can be for either partner.

It also increased the intimacy my partner and I share. If you love your partner, sexual embrace is one of the sexiest and most intense times to say it.

Sex is an expression of your love, so when you are in a sensual position, like missionary, try vocally expressing your feelings. Oxytocin will immediately flood both of your brains, deepening your connection and putting your sex into overdrive.

I noticed that our communication got better as well. We already communicate well about what we like and don't like, but after we started talking during sex, it became easier to openly discuss new things we wanted to try.

This can be tough for many people, because often, the things you want to try in bed may also seem a little weird to you or your partner. They can make you feel uncomfortable just thinking about it. These desires sometimes come from deep within our psyche, where many of our insecurities and past experiences come together.

But, as you gain more comfort talking to each other while having sex, while you're both at your most vulnerable, it makes discussing this stuff outside the bedroom a little easier.

My partner and I started with relatively benign things, like a certain toy we wanted to try but never had before, or a smaller fantasy that would add a different dynamic to our sex.

It escalated from there as we got more comfortable with each other, and as our trust in one another grew and solidified. This unlocked certain fantasies and desires we never knew we had. I think that is one of the coolest byproducts of making sex talk a regular and comfortable habit.

In terms of having sex with both your partner's body and their mind, talking is the absolute best way I have found to tap into the sexual depths of your partner's psyche.

This is when you say stuff like, "Do you like it when I ride you like this?" and they inevitably respond with an enthusiastic "yes" (because you read the tips in the Powerful Positions chapter), it confirms in their *mind* that what is happening to their *body* is amazing.

I know it can seem weird in the beginning. It was a little weird for me as well. But as with any sexual advancement, try your best to keep an open mind to the possibilities before you. And there is no harm in taking things slow and at your own pace.

Often, someone may say they don't like something in the bedroom, but in reality, they just haven't been with someone they like doing it with.

Maybe they think they won't like it before even trying it. So whether it's you or your partner that's apprehensive, put yourself into your partner's shoes, practice some empathy, and develop a platform of trust to build upon.

The following sections detail a number of methods for introducing dirty talk into your sex life.

Sex Talk Should Begin Outside the Bedroom

If you have never talked during sex before, the best time to begin is actually when you are *not* having sex.

Compliment your partner on their butt when they wear tight pants. Tell them that it's sexy when they polish their car. Tell them that it drives you crazy when they wear a certain perfume or cologne.

This primes your minds for more sexual dialogue when the time comes. It creates a constant sexual dynamic between you two that becomes easier to transfer to the bedroom.

At its core, you are flirting with heavy sexual undertones.

As I became more comfortable with my sexuality, in part by having more experience, and in part by reading, I discovered I have a natural tendency for sexual flirtation with my partner. My mind can spot sexual innuendos a mile away (or should I say, in YOUR endos).

It's noticing something that's not inherently sexual, and spinning it in a way that makes it sexual. You can do this as well. All it takes is practice.

Here are some examples:

Your Partner: "I can't believe it's so wet out there!" (when it's raining outside)

You: "I'll make you so wet, in here." (joking, but not really)

Your Partner: "I got such a good workout today."

You: "I hope you saved some energy, because we'll be working out all night."

A sign on the road that says, "$5 CARWASH, FREE LUBE."

You turn to your partner and say, "I know how we could use some free lube."

You get the idea. You're making otherwise random connections into sexual ones. It's fun. It's lighthearted. And it's a good way to introduce sexual dialogue and banter.

When you say the innuendo or pun, say it in a way that is obviously joking rather than serious. Smile. Give your partner a funny look. Chuckle at yourself afterwards and lovingly tap your partner on the arm.

Sex should be fun, so talking about it should be fun as well.

Some Suggested Lines to Try...

Here are some lines that I like to say or hear in bed (or I've heard that other people enjoy).

I broke them up into levels, Level 1 being the least raunchy and easiest to begin with, and Level 3 being the most raunchy.

Level 1-

"I love your [body part]" (This could be their ass, their boobs, their genitals, their feet. Whatever erotic body part you feel inspired to compliment.)

"I love the way you [action]" (This could be the way they ride you, the way they give you oral sex, the way they moan, etc.)

"You are so sexy" or "You are so beautiful" or "You are so hot" or "You are so [compliment]."

"Do you like being [action]-ed by me?"

"Keep going" or "Keep [action]" (When you are really enjoying something your partner is doing. This line is great for when they have found the sweet spot to make you climax.)

"I'm about to come" or "I'm about to come so hard" or "I'm almost there."

"I want your [body part] so badly."

"I am so ready for you."

"You look so good naked."

Try a few of these the next time you have sex and see what happens.

Experiment. Be a sexual scientist.

Level 2-

"Tell me what you want me to do to you."

"I want you to [action] me."

"I love the way you taste" (Great for oral sex or when your partner feels insecure about their genitals.)

"Do you like my [body part] inside you" or "Do you like it when I fuck you with this [toy]."

"Yeah? Say it again" (when you have asked them a question like the one above.)

"I want you to come all over my [body part]."

"I want to come all over your [body part]."

"Turn over" or "[insert command]."

Level 3-

"I'm going to have my way with you."

"I want you to have your way with me".

"Tie me up" or "Hold me down" or "Hold my arms down."

"[*anything that digs deeper into either of your fantasies/fetishes*]"

I know that some of these can seem weird at first, so ease into it with Level 1 stuff. Gradually move up whenever you feel comfortable.

The level of trust between you and your partner is key. Some of these lines can mean completely different things under different contexts.

With anything new you try, pay attention to how your partner reacts afterwards. This will let you know whether to keep doing it, change it up, or to stop. In the best cases, they will flat out tell you.

Of course, there are also certain things you can say in bed that will be turn-offs rather than turn-ons, and that's okay. Don't let it stop you from being vocal. You will know immediately whether it's something you should keep saying or something you should never say again.

You are constantly learning, so don't get down on yourself. Chalk it up to a funny or interesting experience, and then move on with your life (or in this case, your sex life).

You have learned a lot so far. So I think it's time to put it all together.

The next three chapters take everything you've learned and combine them into a full sexual experience.

You have the theory down. Now it's time to apply it.

Chapter 10

THE ART OF THE TRANSITION

Sex is a fluid performance. It's dynamic, flowing from one thing to another.

Or at least, that is what's supposed to happen…

When I first started having sex, my repertoire consisted of three positions: partner on top, missionary, and doggy style. And I usually rotated through them in that same order.

There was no flow. It was just, "Okay, you've been on top for a while. Let's move to missionary. Okay, that's enough of missionary. How about some doggy style? Alright, let's mix it up again with a little missionary."

This doesn't mean it was bad sex. We were both satisfied. But it didn't have the natural flow it could have had, which gives you the fiery, passionate sex that's always raved about.

What was missing from my sex life in the early days was **deliberate transition from one move to another.**

For one, I wasn't comfortable enough to be assertive in my decisions just yet. I also didn't have enough in the memory bank to pull from when it was time to do something else.

All of this came with experience and knowledge, but there is something to be said about consciously understanding The Art of the Transition.

Sexual Flow – Piecing Everything Together

Luckily, you've read everything up until now and should have a good amount of activities to choose from in the bedroom. Let's piece them together into something with sexual flow.

We're going to break this down in a way that isn't necessarily the sexiest possible, but it will make it understandable and actionable.

The typical sexual flow goes something like this:

Foreplay —> Oral Sex —> Sex —> Orgasm(s) —> Come down/refractory period

Of course, one phase or the other is skipped sometimes, and I get that this isn't typical of the entire population. But it's the easiest way for me to explain this concept.

We're going to detail the same general flow, but add much more between "Oral Sex" and "Orgasm(s)."

What have we learned so far that we could add in? What choices do you have?

- **Manual stimulation** of each other's genitals, which you learned during foreplay.
- **Fellatio and cunnilingus**, with each of the variations you can add to them (fingering, working the balls, stimulating the perineum, stimulating the anus, using your hand and fingers in combination with your mouth, kissing the area, teasing, etc).
- **Anal sex.**

- **The Powerful Positions**, including penetrative, non-penetrative, and oral sex positions. The penetrative positions were further broken down to the penetrating partner on top, on bottom, or coming from behind (and of course I included my own position - "Gravity" - for your pleasure, of course).
- **Incorporating sex toys** and how to use them – dildos, vibrators, vibrating rings, and kinky and restrictive devices.
- **And getting vocal in the bedroom** and how it can enhance your sex life.

That's a pretty good list right there, but it's a lot to remember in the heat of the moment. Let's go one-by-one and see how you can incorporate each into some sort of sexual flow.

We're trying to include this stuff between "Oral Sex" and "Orgasm(s)" of this diagram:

Foreplay —> **Oral Sex** —> Sex —> **Orgasm(s)** —> Come down/refractory period

Manual Stimulation-

As you already know, manual stimulation involves using your hand(s) to stimulate your partner. It's a great way to warm each other up during foreplay, **but it can also be done while transitioning from one move to another.**

Imagine you are in a doggy style (receiving partner on hands and knees, penetrating partner from behind) and you have decided to switch to doggy style lying sideways. You can always direct your partner to move into this position and continue on with it.

BUT, you can also add in some manual stimulation.

For example, let's say you have a penis and you don't want to have an orgasm yet, but you are getting very close. You can manually stimulate your partner before going to the next position, to give yourself some time to come down and to keep your partner aroused.

You could also take this opportunity to be more intimate, kissing each other before the next position, or to heighten the kinkiness by saying what you're about to do to each other.

Here are some key places to throw in **manual stimulation** during your sexual flow:

- If you are moving from oral sex on the floor to having sex on the bed, pause to manually stimulate your partner.
- If you're changing positions.
- If your partner orgasms best from manual stimulation, you may want to transition to manual stimulation to make them climax.
- It's possible that you could do manual stimulation as part of the come down period, but usually people's genitals are too sensitive for contact immediately after orgasm. However, manual stimulation can come in handy again once the refractory period is over. If you two are ready for another round, start manually stimulating each other to get things going.

Fellatio and Cunnilingus-

Oral sex is my favorite aspect to throw into the sexual flow. Similar to manual stimulation, I believe it's best done in between different positions.

You can move from a position on the bed, to having one partner on the floor giving oral, to having sex against the wall, to oral sex on the bed, to another position on the bed. The opportunities are endless.

All you need to know is that you have **options** when moving from one thing to another. It mixes it up. It makes sex more mysterious and more spontaneous.

If your partner has a penis, we're generally speaking in terms of fellatio that is a precursor to more sexual activity (Pre-Sex Fellatio).

You're trying to avoid the refractory period for now. If you are the one giving oral, try not to make it overly pleasurable, but it should still feel good. If you are the one receiving, control yourself and stop your partner if you get close to the point of no return (when you are about to come and can't stop yourself).

If your partner has a vagina, it doesn't matter whether you receive oral sex as a precursor to more sexual activity or the sexual activity in and of itself, because the technique is the same either way. You're going for maximum pleasure.

If you are the one giving oral sex, it doesn't mean you should put tons of pressure on yourself to give your partner an orgasm every time you transition into oral sex. For the sake of transitioning and spontaneity, if you end up giving your partner an orgasm (or multiple) that's awesome. But don't shy away from doing it by putting too much pressure on yourself.

How long should you remain in each transition? Unfortunately, I can't give you an totally clear answer. **Enough time to make it worthwhile,** so you are able to give or receive pleasure for a definite period of time, but not long enough so that it halts your momentum.

You're going to have to judge this one yourself. Just know that if you spend too long in a transition, that transition becomes the sexual activity in and of itself, rather than a part of the sexual flow.

Don't bounce around like you're on crack, but don't lag too long in any one transition.

Anal Sex-

Throwing in anal sex can be tricky, but it's doable. The key components here are proper preparation and hygiene.

Depending on the receiving partner, they may need some time to warm up before penetration happens so that it doesn't cause them loads of pain. Some people can go straight for it, but let's assume this isn't the case:

1. Make sure you have lube handy, preferably before starting any sexual activity. Place it within easy reach so you don't have to waste time finding it, especially in the dark.

2. Make sure you have multiple condoms handy. Key word: Multiple. You will see why in a second.

3. You or your partner can do this, but place a condom on your finger, lather it with some lube, and use it to warm your partner up. Get their anus used to being stimulated and penetrated.

4. When you two are ready for penetration, use a different condom for the object doing the penetration, lather it with some lube, and you're on your merry way.

When you are ready to transition into something else, TAKE THE CONDOM OFF.

Sorry, didn't mean to yell at you. But this is important.

You DO NOT want to use the same condom for something else that has just been used for anal sexual activity.

Take it off, throw it away, and you should be good to go. But to be safe, if you want to use the object again in further activity, it may be smart to clean it first.

Using this method, you should be ready to safely add anal sex into your sexual flow whenever you and your partner wish.

The Powerful Positions-

First, a recap of the positions:

Penetrative-

- *#1 Missionary With Legs in the Air*

- *#2 Missionary While Grabbing the Butt*

- *#3 Receiving Partner Sideways and Penetrating Partner On Top*

- *#4 Legs in the Air on Edge of the Bed*
- *#5 Doggy Style With Receiving Partner Curling Towards Other Partner*
- *#6 Doggy Style With Penetrating Partner Squatting Over*
- *#7 From Behind With Receiving Partner Laying On Stomach*
- *#8 Sideways Penetration From Behind*
- *#9 Receiving Partner On Top (with variations)*

Non-Penetrative-

- *#1 Rubbing Together of the Genitals*
- *#2 Mutual Masturbation*

Oral Sex-

- *#1 68-ing (variation of 69)*
- *#2 Fellatio Variations*
- *#3 Cunnilingus Variations*

Michael's Powerful Position-

- *#1 Gravity*

It seems like quite a lot to juggle, but it's not too complicated once we break it down.

If you will notice…

- Numbers 1 through 4 are all with the **penetrating partner on top** and the **receiving partner on bottom**.

- Numbers 5 through 8 are all with the **penetrating partner coming from behind**.

- Number 9 contains a few variations, all with the **receiving partner on top**.

- The non-penetrative positions are straightforward, usually with **both partners lying next to each other**.

- The oral sex positions simply place you in the **best position for both partners to be comfortable and to have access to oral stimulation**.

- And Gravity is straightforward.

All it takes to transition is to decide what *type* of position you want to get into next, then choose a variation.

For instance, say you are in *#4 Legs in the Air on Edge of the Bed* and you want to transition to an oral sex position. If you are the partner receiving oral sex, decide how you want to situate yourself in the room.

Let's say you choose sitting on the bed with your partner on the floor. Simply direct your partner how you want them to be situated, position yourself, and you have successfully transitioned from one powerful position to another.

Let's try another example. Say you want to transition from *#1 Missionary With Legs in the Air* to a position with the receiving partner on top. If you are the receiving partner and you want to be on top, you may direct your partner by either physically suggesting that you want them on their back or telling them that you want to be on top.

From there, you have a number of options. Do you want straddle your partner on your knees while facing them? Do you want to squat over them? Do you want to straddle them and lean backward, placing your hands on their legs for support? Do you want to face the opposite direction?

Once you have decided, you have successfully transitioned from yet another powerful position to another one. It's deceptively simple.

The guideline:

1. Choose a type of position to get into next (i.e. penetrating partner on top, penetrating partner from behind, receiving partner on top, a non-penetrative position, or an oral sex position)
2. Choose a variation
3. Situate yourself in the correct position and direct your partner
4. You're good to go!

If you can remember the types of positions you have available, the variations should come to you naturally while you're having sex.

When you want to switch positions, just ask yourself, "Which *type* of position do I want to get into, and which *variation* do I want to do?"

Incorporating Sex Toys-

To recap, here are our four main types of toys:

- dildos
- vibrators
- vibrating rings
- kinky and restrictive devices

Incorporating sex toys is my second favorite thing to add to the sexual flow. It's extremely exciting when either you or your partner spontaneously busts out a sex toy to use.

Along with getting vocal, this is another quick way to take your sex life to the next level. Just incorporating one sex toy can do the trick. Multiple, and you're a sexual magician.

If you decide to use toys while having sex, the best thing you can do is prepare yourself. This accomplishes two things:

1. You won't interrupt your flow by searching for the toy.
2. You know exactly which ones you have available, making it easier to transition.

How do you prepare yourself?

Choose an area where they won't be disturbed by your activity (they won't jostle around and move out of place) **and where they can be accessed quickly and easily.**

A bedside table is great for this.

Lay out your dildo(s), lube, vibrator(s), vibrating ring(s), and any kinky or restrictive devices you want to use. Try to do this before you start having sex, so they're ready to go when you need them.

Now to transition.

A dildo can be used any time in your sexual flow. Just transition from whatever your position you're in, grab the dildo, and you're off to the races.

A vibrator can be slightly trickier if you want to use it in addition to intercourse. If you're trying to avoid exiting your partner or having your partner exit, which could disrupt your flow, make sure the vibrator is within reach or being held by one partner beforehand.

For a vibrating ring, one of the best places to keep it is on your finger. You can snag it anytime, pop it on, and you're good to go.

Kinky and restrictive devices – these are extremely fun to incorporate as well. When I am in any position, I don't mind completely stopping, going over and grabbing a blindfold, putting it on my partner, and then proceeding after that.

You can incorporate another toy, get into a different position, go for manual stimulation or oral sex, put on a restrictive device without them knowing – whatever your mind can come up with. This is your chance to become creative.

And if you want to be constrained or have the kinky device used on you, don't be shy about letting your partner know. Use one of the lines in the chapter on getting vocal to make your request in a hot and sexual way.

With toys, the more you use them, the more your mind will naturally work to find new ways to incorporate them into your sex life.

Getting Vocal in the Bedroom-

First off, you do not need to wait for a transition to be vocal. You can talk any time you want. However, being vocal *while* you're transitioning can really enhance the transition itself.

If you are thinking about using a toy on your partner, go ahead and tell them what you're about to do. Then do it.

If you want your partner to penetrate you a certain way, tell them the way you want them to enter you, and you two will be scrambling as fast as you can to get into that position.

If you love the way your partner tastes and you want to give them oral, tell them that, and then transition into it.

Use your words to intensify the moment. That's what they are there for.

Getting Comfortable With Deliberate Decision Making

Whether you are the more dominant or submissive partner, it's important to get comfortable making deliberate decisions about what you want to do in bed.

Move through your transitions with conviction. Sex only takes a standstill once the mind stops working. So keep your mind active, and make those decisions deliberately.

A Final Note on Transitioning

In its essence, the exact transition through sexual flow comes naturally depending on the partners. But having the background knowledge above should open your options immensely and give you some great ways to apply everything we have been discussing so far.

Just to clarify, do not feel like you need to follow everything I say exactly.

This is a *guide* to having great sex. The way you wish to have sex is ultimately up to you.

But use the knowledge in this book to find the way YOU love to have sex, and how you can make it the best experience possible for you and your partner.

Chapter 11

DEVELOPING SEXUAL INTUITION

Sexual intuition is when you instinctively know *what* you want to do next in the bedroom and *how* to do it.

Sexual intuition has a close relationship with The Art of the Transition. As you gain a deeper understanding of transitioning, which transitions work best, and the way you and your partner enjoy doing them, sexual intuition develops.

You don't have to think about what to do next. You just do it.

You don't have to think about placing toys within reach. You just do it.

You don't have to think about what to say to your partner during sex. When the time is right, the right sentence comes out of your mouth and changes the whole dynamic.

It involves taking all of the information that has been discussed so far, applying it to your sex life, experiencing it first hand, molding it into your own unique style, and making it a habit.

You *naturally* progress through the sexual flow. Your creativity in the bedroom becomes natural. Your mind goes into a sexual zone *where thought doesn't have to precede action anymore.*

You and your partner simply exist in the moment, letting nature take over.

It's a beautiful thing.

How Sexual Intuition Develops

Besides applying the information in this book, sexual intuition develops a number of ways.

First, it develops through experience.

I'm guessing that 100% naturals do exist who have sexual intuition the night they lose their virginity (I was not one of them), but I'm also guessing they are a minority. For the rest of us, it's impossible to have sexual intuition without gaining the experience that sex provides.

This is perfectly fine and totally natural. Sexual intuition is not a goal and it is not a destination. It's a byproduct of taking an active interest in your sex life and continuously learning along the way.

It's a byproduct of having fun, making mistakes, learning from them, and trying new things. It's a part of the experience.

Second, it develops through communication.

Communication deepens the connection between two people. It opens the doors to each other's desires and fantasies. Once you know these fantasies, you can learn how to tap into them in different ways.

If your partner has a fantasy of being constrained, you can tap into that physically and mentally. If they have a desire to be dominant, you can tap into that fantasy by playing the submissive role.

Third, sexual intuition develops through sexual compatibility.

We will be discussing sexual compatibility in a later chapter, but it boils down to how well your sexual desires, biology, and values fit together with your partner.

I have had partners where the sex was terrible, not because either of us was "bad" in bed, but because we weren't compatible with each other.

I loved doing something, like pulling hair, and my partner hated it. I didn't like something, like getting my ass slapped, and my partner loved it. Sometimes the flow was completely off. Sometimes we weren't fully comfortable with each other and it made things awkward. This stuff happens, and it is neither partner's fault. It simply is, and neither of you have much control over it.

But when you ARE compatible, that's when things get interesting. That's when sex starts to happen naturally. It progresses seemingly without any mental effort. And as you continue to experience more and more together, the sexual intuition you have with each other grows further.

The Right Way to Think About Sexual Intuition

Don't make it your goal to "achieve" sexual intuition. You will know when you experience it.

Instead, focus on having fun, first and foremost. Then focus on the connection your have with your partner or partners. Then focus on being open minded, trying new things, experimenting, unlocking sexual fantasies and desires, and sharing this awesome experience of human connection together.

Sexual intuition is a byproduct of leading a pure sex life, one that isn't revolved around ego fulfillment or manipulation, but around genuine caring for another person and the joy felt when giving them pleasure and receiving it yourself.

Chapter 12

MASTERING MULTITASKING

Welcome to the Tips and Tricks chapter! I know this is the one you have all been waiting for.

There is where we talk about the subtle pleasurable acts that lead to HUGE differences in the bedroom. You can do some of these just about any time during sex and some are situational, but all are fun and easy to implement.

They are:

- Scratching
- Ass slapping
- Biting
- Nibbling
- Hair pulling (and hair constraining)
- Breathing into their ear
- More manual stimulation
- Sucking
- Covering their eyes
- Grabbing body parts
- Constraining body parts

- Pretend choking

I'm calling this "Multitasking" because more often than not, you wouldn't be doing these things without some sort of other sexual activity as well.

Usually, they are done in conjunction with something else, like fellatio, intercourse, cunnilingus, foreplay, or during a transition. So while they *can* be done by themselves, I feel that it's more useful to describe them in ways that help you multitask.

Multitasking also provides extra points of stimulation other than the genitals. It creates a more total body dynamic when having sex.

You *could* just do missionary, but sucking on your partner's neck at the same time, or having your partner suck on your neck, adds more to it. You *could* just do doggy style with your partner curling towards you, or you could do it while slapping your partner's ass every once in a while or having your partner slap your ass.

It's more exciting, and it's simple to implement once you understand your options.

I multitask almost constantly. I'm almost never doing just one thing at a time. I always trying to combine the main activity with something that I know my partner enjoys (because we have talked about what each other likes and doesn't like).

Whenever I try something new, afterwards I'll either ask her how she felt about it, or if she beats me to it, she'll tell me straight away.

Let's go over some ways to implement multitasking into your sexual flow.

Scratching-

Scratching is an awesome one to try. It adds just the right amount of pain to the pleasure, and it adds a little more kinkiness.

If you are on bottom in a missionary type position, try reaching up and scratching down the entire expanse of your partner's back. This feels good and lets them know that you're impressed with their skills on top.

If you are the penetrating partner in a doggy style position (coming from behind), your partner's back should be exposed in front of you. Give it a good scratch. They won't know it's coming, and it will send tingles down their back afterwards.

Scratching is also nice to add during foreplay when you want to heighten arousal. Or during oral sex, to give them an extra touchpoint of pleasure by scratching down the sides of their legs or arms.

However, be careful not to break the skin. (Unless you're into that.)

Ass Slapping-

Slapping dat ass!

Ass slapping is a fun way to kink up your sex life. Doggy style positions are the best positions I have found to incorporate this multitasking technique. You can also do it during transitions as you are getting into another position or moving to oral sex.

Butts are pretty padded, so it should be able to take a good slap. This is a common one during sex, so if you don't like it, you may want to let your partner know beforehand.

If you do like it, and you want your ass slapped, go ahead and tell your partner while having sex. They should be more than happy to satisfy that desire for you.

Biting-

By biting, I don't mean biting so hard that you break the skin. Just like scratching or ass slapping, I suggest adding just enough pain so that it doesn't override the pleasure.

Some people hate being bitten (I know a few people), so proceed with caution and pay attention to how your partner reacts.

Good places to bite are the more meaty areas – thighs, shoulders, neck, arms, etc.

In general, you don't want to do this randomly, but while your partner is being stimulated at the same time. (That's a good rule to follow for almost all of these.)

Nibbling-

Nibbling means a slight bite with the front champers, not an entire mouth ordeal. It's just an extra bit of stimulation on a sensitive area.

Try the ear lobes. The ears are surprisingly sensual. You can also try nibbling on their lips and nipples.

Hair Pulling (and hair constraining)-

When hair is pulled, it stimulates the hair follicles, which can feel especially good while your genitals are being stimulated.

In general, you don't want to pull a small amount of your partner's hair. This will hurt. Grab a sizable chunk and give it a tug.

Don't attempt to rip it out, but pull it enough so that there is tension on the hair follicles. Depending on the position, their head may actually bend backwards.

Hair pulling is most common during doggy style positions. You can also restrain your partner during missionary type positions by holding their hair down on the bed.

Breathing in their ear-

Don't do this one excessively, but every once in a while it can feel *really* good.

Lean your head near your partner's ear, and give them one slow, sensual breath that hits the general area. The ear is a sensual organ, so your partner may respond with pleasurable shudders down their spine.

More manual stimulation-

Manual stimulation can also be a part of multitasking.

If your partner has a vagina, just about any position where you can reach the clitoris is a good opportunity to try stimulating it with your thumb or fingers, as long as it isn't too sensitive. You will know once you give it a try.

If your partner has a penis and testicles, just about any position where you can reach either one is a good opportunity to try stimulating them as well.

You can also stimulate the outer part of the anus or insert a finger to stimulate the inner part, if your partner enjoys it.

Sucking-

Sucking on different parts of my partner's body is one of my favorite ways to multitask. It provides a good balance between pain and pleasure.

You can suck on your partner's neck (a highly erogenous zone), AKA give them a hickie. It may have a bad reputation, as if you're marking your territory (because of the possible bruise). But it feels good nonetheless.

You can also suck on your partner's nipples, which can be sensitive to stimulation and provide a lot of pleasure. And on their fingers, toes, or ear lobe.

Covering your partner's eyes-

This is something I like to do if I don't have a blindfold available, or if I don't want to pause having sex to get it.

Simply take your hand and cover their eyes as you're having sex.

Once again, it adds a sense of mystery for your partner and gives you a sense of domination, or the other way around if you are the partner getting your eyes covered.

A great time to do this is during missionary type positions, during doggy style lying on your sides, or while giving oral sex if you can reach far enough.

Grabbing, holding, and stimulating body parts-

You heard me talk about "leverage" quite a lot in the chapter on positions. It's when you're holding onto something to help aid in thrusting or sexual motion.

There are a few parts of your partner's body that are useful for this. You can grab your partner's arms, especially if you are in a position where the penetrating partner is coming from behind, or if you are in a missionary type position.

If your partner has breasts, grabbing them can provide leverage for you and pleasure for them. If you have breasts, grabbing your own and massaging them can also be very erotic for your partner to see.

Grabbing hold of your partner's butt is another good one. Try giving them an ass slap and grabbing it right afterwards.

You can also up the intimacy by holding hands with your partner while having sex.

Constraining body parts-

Constraining parts of your partner's body is similar to grabbing and holding onto them, but with the specific purpose of restricting movement.

If you are on top in a missionary style position, you can hold your partner's arms down. If you are coming from behind, you can grab your partner's arms and hold them backward. You can also grab your partner's hands and hold them down, constraining them and keeping you balanced and stable at the same time.

If you are providing oral sex, try constraining your partner's legs.

Pretend choking-

You must be very careful with this one, and I suggest discussing it with your partner before trying it. Also, come up with a safety action to let your partner know if you ever want to stop, like tapping their shoulder 3 times or tapping them on the nose. Make it something obvious.

Choking is a dominant act, and must be done with a high level of trust between both partners. You don't want to entirely constrict the airway.

You want to give their mind the *perception* of being choked, so apply most of the pressure to the sides of the neck where their muscles are, rather than on the front where the windpipes are located.

If your partner is doing it to you, make sure to tell them how you would like it to be done.

Again, communication and safety are important here. But it can be an extremely hot way to multitask, if done in the right environment.

Mastering Multitasking

You are completely free to be creative here. Combine as many of these as you wish, and try to come up with some new ones that I haven't covered.

It may seem daunting at first to see this list, so when you know you are going to have sex, pick one or two and implement them. Then communicate with your partner afterwards and see if they liked them. Once you get comfortable, move on to more.

Soon enough, they will become a natural part of your sexual flow, and you will have become a master of multitasking.

As you try certain moves in the bedroom, you will notice that each has a level of dominance and submission associated with it.

These roles play out constantly in the bedroom. The next chapter tells you how this happens, and how to take advantage of it in your sex life.

Chapter 13

THE BALANCE OF DOMINANCE

I have mentioned dominance and submission several times. Now it's time to explain it.

Once you know your options in the bedroom, it's a good time to play around with the balance of dominance.

I am the more dominant partner in my sex life, but I wasn't always like this. In the beginning, I was usually more passive or on the same level as my partner. This meant that I wasn't making very many decisions, I wasn't directing the sexual flow, and I wasn't taking any sort of control, like constraining or restricting my partner.

As I became more comfortable in the bedroom, my true sexuality started to come out. I naturally grew into the more dominant partner, and I was more sexually compatible with partners that leaned towards the submissive side of the spectrum.

This lead to some great sex, but also some not-so-great sex when I ended up with partners that were dominant as well.

My view is, when two submissive partners or two dominant partners have sex, one has to secede and one has to take the reigns as the more dominant partner, even if the balance is only slightly skewed.

This means that for the most part, one has to follow the directions of the other and one has to give directions. I may be totally wrong here in many instances, but in general, this is what I believe is true.

You will have to decide what's true in your own sex life. For now, it's important to note that this aspect of sex *does* exist and it plays out in noticeable ways.

Characteristics of the Dominant Partner

Here are some potential characteristics of the more dominant partner:

- They make decisions in the bedroom, such as what to transition to and how to do it.

- They do more of the constricting and constraining – exercising control.

- They usually use toys on their partner, rather than the other way around.

- They usually initiate the use of toys on themselves by commanding or suggesting that their partner do so.

- They are usually more focused on their partner's pleasure, rather than their partner focusing on them (the keyword here is "more." I'm not saying this definitively, but this is how the spectrum is generally oriented).

- They are usually more vocal in telling their partner what they are going to do next.

- They are usually the partner doing more things to their partner, rather than their partner doing things to them.

- They usually initiate sex more often.

- They tap into the submissiveness of their partner, giving more commands than requests.

- They usually take more responsibility for their partner's pleasure and orgasms.

Characteristics of the Submissive Partner

Here are some potential characteristics of the more submissive partner:

- They follow more direction rather than giving it.

- They vocally confirm what their partner is doing to them.

- They typically don't make commands, but rather request what they want to do and how they want to be pleasured.

- They mostly have toys used on them, rather than initiating the use of toys on their partner.

- They are usually the recipient of most of the physical pleasure.

- They are usually subject to the sexual flow, rather than directing it.

- They typically initiate sex less often, and enjoy when their partner initiates it.

- They tap into the dominance of their partner, releasing control.

Of course, these are all generalities and are not meant to be taken as matter of fact statements. Everyone's balance is different, and it fluctuates with different partners who have different compatibilities with each other. It also fluctuates as you gain more experience in the bedroom, as it did with me.

Hopefully, you can now identify where you and your partner(s) lie on the spectrum. Once you understand this, you can orient your sex more towards the end of the spectrum you are on.

And when you're having sex and going through the sexual flow, you will be able to tell whether you should be more dominant or submissive depending on what's happening.

How to Apply the Balance of Dominance to Your Sexual Communication

The balance of dominance can cause some conflict in the bedroom, especially when partners are new to each other and haven't figured out each other's sexual tendencies yet.

Let's say you are a very dominant partner, and your partner is slightly submissive. You express your dominance through ass slapping, directing the sexual flow by physically suggesting which positions to get into, and you enjoy pretend choking.

Your partner enjoys being submissive by getting their ass slapped and by following your direction, but being choked is too dominant and makes your partner feel uncomfortable.

If this hasn't been communicated beforehand, this could lead to trying out choking for the first time and receiving a defensive response from your partner.

Obviously, you will respect their wishes to not be choked, but you may feel that some of your dominance has been undermined, making you feel less like yourself in the bedroom. And your partner may feel like they didn't play their usual role, and may feel like the sex is off.

This is one of the reasons why communication is so important. Often, the things we like and dislike in the bedroom have dominant or submissive characteristics attached to them, as in the above case. Some examples:

- Doing the ass slapping – perceived as more dominant
- Getting their ass slapped – perceived as more submissive
- Directing the sexual flow – perceived as more dominant
- Following the direction – perceived as more submissive
- Doing the pretend choking – perceived as more dominant
- Being choked – perceived as more submissive

When these likes and dislikes aren't communicated properly, it can lead to conflict and a disruption of the dominance/submission balance.

When discussing the intricacies of your sex life with your partner, pay attention to the dominant and submissive characteristics of each act. It may give you some insight as to why your partner dislikes or likes something, and to the nature of your own desires.

It also becomes easier to make requests in the bedroom, like when you want to try something new that your partner isn't comfortable with. They may be more open to trying it if they understand that it's coming from your desire to be dominant or submissive, and you may be more open to trying what your partner wants to do if you understand where their desires are coming from.

It also provides a platform from which to tap into your partner's fantasies. You will start finding ways to enhance their dominant or submissive tendencies with subtle things like whispering a certain line in their ear or the way you pull their hair or hold their hands down.

The balance of dominance is fun to play around with and can enhance your communication and understanding of each other.

Which segues into our next chapter perfectly – practicing effective and empathetic communication.

Chapter 14

COMMUNICATION PRACTICES

The absolute greatest sex – by far – happens between two people who care about each other's pleasure equally and unselfishly.

If you want to have great sex, throw out your ego, throw out any self-absorption you have in your sex life, and throw out any sexual selfishness.

Communication must begin from a place of mutual caring for each other's pleasure and satisfaction, from a place of vulnerability, and most importantly, from a place of trust. Only from there can one's sex life reach astronomical heights.

Communication is harped on constantly in sex articles on the internet. But they rarely go farther than, "You should communicate with your partner about what you like and don't like, and be attentive to your partner's needs." While this is true, it goes much deeper than that.

Having sex is one of the most vulnerable acts you can do with another person. All of your insecurities, all of your anxieties, all of your stress about your performance, your body image, your past experiences – they can all converge in the bedroom.

When communicating with your partner, try your best to practice empathy. Try your best to put yourself in their shoes and see things from their perspective. And if they aren't doing this for you, let them know that you would like them to.

It's also important to set up boundaries in the bedroom, especially when you get deeper into sexual fantasies and the kinkier stuff. It takes a long time to build trust in one another, so that trust should be held sacred.

Here's a comment from a Redditor that applies to this topic:

"Trust in the bedroom builds up over time and can be taken away in a second. Define what trust means in and out of the bedroom."

And another Redditor talking about discussing sex with your partner:

"Also, I think that some people may experience awkwardness talking about sex. It's not always easy to discuss casually, we're so afraid of hurting people's feelings or feeling judged."

I think both of these comments hold true.

You may want to tell your partner that you don't like something they've been doing in bed for months, but you haven't had the heart to hurt their feelings. You have decided to keep it inside, but it's becoming a bigger and bigger issue for you. It's hard to bring these things up with someone you care about, and even more difficult to say it in a way that doesn't hurt their feelings.

You may also want to try something new, but this "something" has been deemed "weirder" by societal standards or is not as common, making you feel like you can't talk about it. But it has been eating away at your thoughts and your fantasies. You want to discuss trying it with your partner. You just don't know how. You don't want them to judge you.

I have laid out exact scripts and worksheets you can use to work through this communication with your partner. I'm framing them in a letter format because going through dialogue wouldn't provide as good of an example.

You can use these as samples or follow them exactly. Either way, they should help ease the process. I have also included some helpful considerations to keep in mind when discussing these issues.

Script #1 – Discussing Something You Want to Try

There's something I've been meaning to talk to you about, but I've been holding off on it because it makes me feel a little uncomfortable. I'm more comfortable with you than I have been with anyone else, so I'm going to push through and say it anyway.

It's about something I've been wanting to try in the bedroom. It's not exactly something that our friends have done, and it makes me feel weird just thinking about it. But it has been eating away at my thoughts and I can't keep it in any longer. And most importantly, I want to try it with you, because I trust you so much and my feelings for you are so strong.

I want to try being handcuffed *(note: or whatever you want to try)*. I know you're not into being dominant, but I would love for you have total control over me in the bedroom, at least once, just to see how it is. If you do this for me, I would love to do something for you as well. It'll be like a trade!

Either way, if you are absolutely not comfortable with it, that is totally fine. I don't want you to feel pressured into it, and I wouldn't want to feel that way myself. But I do think it would be something fun to try. If we end up hating it, we can stop immediately. And if we end up loving it, awesome!

Let me know what you think.

Keep in mind-

- Your partner may be uncomfortable with what you want to try, so communicate that you understand this.

- Let them know this isn't something you want to do with just anyone, but that you want to share it with them and them alone (I get that this won't be totally true all the time, but it makes it more special).

- Try to see your request from your partner's perspective, and be empathetic to how they may feel about it.

- Don't pressure them. The more you pressure them, the easier it will be for them to deny your request and more conflict will arise. Give them a way out by saying if they're too uncomfortable, it's okay and it won't change the relationship.

- If your partner is making this type of request to you, imagine that you had a burning desire to try something. Step into your partner's shoes. Think about how you would want your partner to react. Then react accordingly.

Script #2 – Telling Your Partner That You Don't Like Something They Do in Bed

Our sex life is absolutely amazing. You're a freak in bed and you turn me on so much. I get horny just thinking about you as I go about my day.

I love everything you do in bed, especially when you pull my hips into you whenever we have sex *(or whatever you genuinely love about what they do)*. But there's just one thing that I know you like to do, and it's really hot, but it actually kind of hurts me *(or the reason why you don't like it)*.

I wish it didn't, but I can't control it. And I don't want you to feel bad thinking that it's your fault or anything. It's something neither of us can control.

When we're in that position where you're on top of me, and you roll your hips side to side, it feels really good for the most part, except it hurts my lower back quite a lot. I think it's from an old injury I got in high school, but it's pretty painful.

I don't mean to make you feel bad, because if it wasn't for my back, I would love it 100%. You look so hot when you're rolling your hips like that. But it hurts enough to where it totally distracts me from your sexiness.

I know I can't be a complete saint, so if there is anything I'm doing that you don't like, feel free to tell me. I'd rather both of us openly communicate like this and get these things out of the way, than stay silent doing things in the bedroom that actually hinder our sex life.

Keep in mind-

- Your partner may love doing the thing you don't like, and may think that you love it as well. If this is the case, some of their sexual ego and self-esteem may be tied to this act. So let them know the reason(s) why you don't like it, as gently as you can.

- Compliment them on the things you like first. Make them genuine comments. There's no use in communication if you are going to lie and fabricate things. Be honest, but be tactful in your honesty.

- Extend the lines of communication by being open to finding out something they don't like which you do in bed. This makes it more of an open forum, rather than one person being targeted.

Script #3 – Discussing a Fantasy You Have

This is something I have never shared with anyone. I only think about this when I am by myself, and I've kept it a secret for years.

But I want to share it with you, because I trust you not to judge me, even if you don't want to try it.

I have this sexual fantasy. It feels weird for me to actually explain it out loud, so please, don't make fun of me. It's a fantasy where you knock on the front door and pretend like you're delivering a package *(insert whatever fantasy you have)*. We don't know each other, but when we see each other, we're immediately attracted to one another.

You say it's hot outside, so I invite you in for a drink. But next thing I know, you grab my face, pull it in to yours, we start kissing, and eventually stumble into the bedroom and have sex.

I know it sounds a little funny, and it's not like I would want something like that to happen in real life. But I feel so comfortable with you, so pretending like we didn't know each other would be really hot for me.

How do you feel about it?

I also want you to feel comfortable telling me any fantasies you have that you would like to act out. We might as well get them all out in the open and see which ones we want to try. I think it could be really fun. What do you say?

Keep in mind-

- Fantasies can be uncomfortable to discuss, whether they are your own or your partner's. However, they are also completely natural. Pretty much everyone has them. So try to create an environment of understanding in which to let them out.

- Invite your partner to share their fantasies as well.

Script #4 – Talking About Your Insecurities and Anxieties

I wish this didn't bother me, but I can't help it. I feel really insecure about it and it makes me extremely anxious. It's got to do with something we do in the bedroom.

Up until now, I haven't said anything. I know I should have said something in the beginning, and that's my mistake, but I didn't want you to feel like I was taking something away from you. I also know that it's my insecurity and I have to deal with it myself, but it's gotten to a point where I can't do it anymore – at least not for a while until I work through it.

Using the dildo on you makes me very uncomfortable. It's bigger than me, and I'm scared you might like it more than me. I know this is crazy, because that thing is a piece of rubber. But I can't help it. Every time we use it, it makes me feel so uncomfortable.

I know that it's something you enjoy, and to think that a toy could replace me is nuts. But it's an insecurity I have been dealing with my whole life. I hope you can understand that.

I am totally open to other toys, so if there is something else you want to try in the meantime, I'm all ears. I just can't use that one anymore. I'll get through it eventually, but for now, it's causing me too much stress.

Thanks for being so understanding. If you have something you would like to talk about, I promise I won't judge you either and I'll do my best to help you through it.

Keep in mind-

- Insecurities run deep. They can cause people intense amounts of stress and anxiety, especially when it comes to sex.

- In the present, insecurities are largely uncontrollable. It takes time to work through these things. So if your partner suddenly brings up something they would like to stop doing in bed, don't take it personally. This may be something they have been dealing with for years, and it may have been hard to talk to you about it.

- Also, don't be afraid to express your insecurities. Often, one of the best ways to get through them is simply to let them out. Tell them to someone you trust and who cares about you. They may be able to provide a different perspective to help you out.

- Once again, maintain an open forum. When expressing an insecurity, your partner may be harboring their own. Give them an opportunity to express theirs as well so you can work through each other's together.

Establishing Boundaries

Knowing each other's boundaries is an essential part of communication. This is where you really get to know your partner's likes, dislikes, and subtle sexual tendencies. These play out in the bedroom constantly, so it's important that you're attentive to them.

I understand this is harder to do with casual relationships and one-night stands. Sometimes the nature of the relationship dictates that this stuff isn't communicated.

What you can do is a simplified version of what I'm about to show you. You would do everything verbally, and usually right after or right before having sex. Then, if you end up having sex again, you will understand much more about your partner's desires, your partner will understand much more about your own, and it will materialize itself into better sex.

I got this idea from a commenter on Reddit. The commenter noted that when she first got together with her partner of 10 years, she wrote out a list of things for them to discuss about their sex life. Each item was rated on a scale of 1-10. Afterwards, they could swap papers, compare answers, and have a much more open and structured discussion about their sex life.

They also came up with a sexual bucket list, which can give partners goals to strive for and make trying new things more fun. I think both of these ideas are brilliant.

Using these two ideas, you can gain a number of things:

- Knowledge of what your partner likes and dislikes.
- What boundaries you should stick to.
- A platform for open communication.
- Goals to work towards together.
- A way to communicate without actually having to say anything, which can make it easier to get started.

I've come up with two sample lists, one including topics for discussion where you would provide a rating for each, and another with possible goals for a sexual bucket list.

I suggest using these as a guide, creating your own, and trying them out. You never know how much it could deepen your connection and improve your communication skills.

Topics for discussion (the first four came from the Redditor)-

1. What level of trust do you have for your partner in the bedroom?
2. How kinky are you?
3. How kinky do you think your partner is?
4. How kinky are you willing to go for your partner?
5. How comfortable are you talking openly about sex?
6. How much do you enjoy giving oral sex?
7. How much do you enjoy receiving oral sex?
8. How much foreplay do you like, 1 being "not very much" and 10 being "a lot"?
9. How willing are you to try anal sex?
10. How willing are you to try having sex in public?
11. How willing are you to try experimenting with sex toys?
12. How comfortable do you feel with being vocal in the bedroom?
13. How comfortable do you feel being constrained by your partner?
14. How comfortable do you feel being blindfolded?
15. How comfortable do you feel watching porn with your partner?
16. How comfortable are you discussing sexual fantasies?
17. How comfortable are you acting out sexual fantasies?

18. How much do you enjoy being more dominant?

19. How much do you enjoy being more submissive?

20. How much do you struggle with sexual anxiety and insecurity?

When you print it out, write a number from 1 to 10 next to each question. Each partner should fill out their own answer sheet.

Afterwards, switch papers and read over your partner's answers. Then discuss each answer. Along the way, you will figure out where your partner's boundaries lie and where to go from there.

Example Sexual Bucket List-

- Have sex on the beach

- Perform oral sex while driving

- Have sex in the backseat of a car

- Have sex on the kitchen floor

- Use a toy on each other at the same time

- Take a trip to the sex shop together

- Watch porn together

- Play a sexual card game

- Have sex four times in one day (or as many as you desire)

- Have sex in the shower

- Perform/receive oral sex in the shower
- Have sex with the curtains open
- Have sex while watching a movie
- Read an erotic book together
- Try constraining each other
- Fulfill one fantasy of each partner
- Research tantric sex together
- Try five new positions every month
- Have anal sex
- Surprise one another with a sexual gift
- Add multitasking into the bedroom
- Have a threesome
- Try switching dominant and submissive roles
- Have sex in every room of the house
- Have sex every day for a month straight
- Have morning sex every day before work for a month straight
- Have sex while cooking dinner

- Have sex while eating dinner

- Make a porno together

Each partner would create their own, switch with their partner, then collaborate with each other on what they want to pursue.

Applying the Communication Principles

The biggest part of communication is practicing empathy. You have to try your best to see where your partner is coming from, and they should do the same for you.

The next big thing is being open and honest with your partner. It's okay if you feel uncomfortable. These things are inherently uncomfortable, but that's why it is so important to talk about them.

Bottling up these thoughts and feelings doesn't do you any good.

Expressing them does you a world of good and will bring you and your partner closer together. You may also experience some of the craziest sex of your life. And all you had to do was tell your partner you wanted to try something new.

Communicate with empathy, communicate honestly and openly, establish boundaries, and write out your desires.

Ba da bing, ba da boom.

Great sex awaits.

Chapter 15

UNLOCKING SEXUAL FANTASIES AND FETISHES

You probably have fantasies and fetishes you don't even know about.

They are lodged in there, in the deeper reaches of your subconscious, and simply haven't had a chance to expose themselves yet.

When I first started having sex, and for about a year and half after, I had no clue I had a fantasy to dominate my partner. I didn't even know what that meant until it happened.

I didn't know that I would find it really hot to tie my partner up, and that my partner would find it really hot as well.

I didn't know that the thrill of getting caught while having sex in public would consume my thoughts for a period of time.

At this point in time, I don't have any strong role playing fantasies. But I am completely open to them, even though my acting skills are crap.

And who knows, maybe I do have a powerful role playing fantasy lodged in there somewhere. There's only one way to find out. I've got to try it.

So, how do fantasies arise out of our subconscious?

I have a theory that a lot of them come from the sexual ideas we were subject to when we were growing up.

I watched a lot of porn in my pubescent days, and as you watch more and more of it, you start going deeper and deeper into the rabbit hole. That may have had an impact on my sexual psyche, and I wouldn't be surprised if it's the same for many people.

If you grew up in a sexually closed off environment, where you were shamed for expressing your sexuality, you may have been compelled to rebel against it, becoming more open-minded and experimental in the process. So the experiences you had in your early sexual development may have had an impact on the fantasies and fetishes you have today.

If you can observe the fantasies you have today, try looking into your past and see if you can find their roots. It may help you understand why you have them, and in turn, help you understand your partner's fantasies and fetishes.

So, if fantasies reside in our subconscious, how do we unlock them?

I believe that the key to unlock these fantasies is made out of the trust you have in one another.

As this trust builds, your mind relaxes, opening the doors to many things (sexual and non-sexual) that allow themselves to be expressed.

It may come in the form of a desire being blurted out randomly in the middle of a sexual conversation. It may come out after a few drinks and your words are flowing out more comfortably than usual. It may come out in the middle of passionate sex, when one of you screams out exactly what they want to be done do them.

This trust leads to opening up to one another, and can be sped up like crazy by following the communication principles presented in the previous chapter.

As you become more comfortable having sexual conversations, that feeling of weirdness starts to go away. Discussing where you want to eat dinner and discussing a new sex toy you want to try become just as natural to talk about.

For those in casual relationships, you start to initiate these conversations more frequently with people you're attracted to, naturally filtering out the people who aren't comfortable discussing it, and naturally filtering in the people who are comfortable. This leads to increased overall sexual compatibility and openness.

These sexual conversations lead you two into the deeper reaches of your desires.

Maybe there's a fantasy you've masturbated to a few times. You begin considering asking your partner if they want to try it. You are a little bit uncomfortable because it's only something you have fantasized about. You have never considered actually making it a reality.

But you and your partner have become so much more comfortable discussing this stuff that it doesn't seem nearly as strange as it would have a while back. So you say, "What the hell, why not? Let's see where this thing takes us."

And so you discuss it, you find out that your partner has fantasized about the exact same thing. Suddenly, you both get that feeling of nervous excitement in the pit of your belly telling you that you're about to have another pivotal experience.

As you share more sexual experiences, the connection grows further. Every experience becomes your little secret that only you two have intimate knowledge about.

This permeates your connection in many ways, through inside jokes as you walk down the street, through a quick glance when someone says something related to your experience together, and through the subtleties of your sexual flow in the bedroom.

All of these things can compound upon each other, leading to spontaneous expressions of these fantasies and fetishes in the bedroom. Without any sort of premeditation, you suddenly get a desire that you've never had before.

You are naturally submissive, but at this moment in time, all you want to do is dominate them.

You have never told your partner how you want to be touched before, but you've suddenly got this unrelenting urge to be touched a certain way, so you whisper it in their ear and make it happen.

These fantasies and fetishes act like little mysteries of the subconscious. Clues pop up all around until in one instant the solution reveals itself and the mystery is solved.

It's an interesting area of sexuality to navigate. There are tons of fantasies and fetishes to choose from (well, I guess in most cases, it's not really a choice). Just go to a porn site and look at the categories. Almost every one of them is a different fantasy or fetish.

I have provided a list of these fantasies and fetishes to show you what is available, and to possibly help you realize that the ones you hold, the ones you feel the most uncomfortable about, are actually quite normal to have.

I would assume that you are certainly not the only one in the world that has this fetish. But if you are, good for you! You can be a trendsetter. There is really no reason to be ashamed of these fantasies.

If you are with a person you trust and who trusts you back, if you have solid communication going on, and if you have become more and more comfortable discussing your sex life and have shared sexual experiences, you should be in a more than ideal environment to express these desires.

Here is a list of some of the more prominent sexual fantasies and fetishes I could find. Just going through this list might unlock something for you.

- Anal sex
- Anal play
- Bondage
- BDSM (Bondage and Sadomasochism)

- Pretending you're strangers meeting each other and going home together
- Teacher and student
- Prisoner and prison guard
- Doctor and patient
- Nurse and patient
- Maid or house cleaner
- Having sex with a coworker
- Having sex with someone you have just met
- Having sex with someone older than you
- Having sex with someone younger than you (of legal age, of course)
- Having sex with multiple people at the same time
- Being completely submissive
- Being completely dominant
- Striptease
- MILFs
- Watching other people have sex
- Squirting
- Having sex on an airplane
- Orgies

- Voyeur (being watched while having sex)
- Different nationalities
- Sexy lingerie
- Gangbang
- Masturbation
- Being sexual with someone that wouldn't constitute a part of your chosen sexual orientation
- Using toys
- Filming each other
- Anilingus
- Footjobs and feet
- Dressing up in school uniforms
- Cheerleader fantasy
- Playing cop and criminal
- Hooking up with the delivery person
- Having sex in public
- Being spanked
- Thrusting into your partner's mouth
- Golden shower (peeing)
- Gagging
- Femdom (feminine domination)

- Fisting
- Deepthroating
- Talking dirty

Odds are, reading some of those may have made you feel uncomfortable. That's alright, especially if you haven't heard of them before.

Don't be judgmental, of yourself or others. It's next to impossible to control what we desire. If your partner expresses something to you that you don't feel comfortable with, react tactfully. If you don't, you could hurt them and tarnish all of the trust you have built together.

Talking About Sexual Fantasies and Fetishes

When discussing these things, use the same model we used in the previous chapter on communication.

You can sit down with your partner, write down all of the fantasies you have and would like to try, then trade papers and compare. It's usually much easier to start out communicating this way than to jump straight into a conversation about it.

But if you're comfortable enough, by all means, don't shy away from having that conversation.

Chapter 16

OVERCOMING SEXUAL ANXIETY AND INSECURITY

Why You're Not Alone In The Bedroom (Hint: It's Not What You Think)

You may feel...

- nervous right before having sex, wondering if your member is going to show up for the game today.

- self-conscious about your body, constantly wondering what your partner is thinking.

- worried that you won't be able to give your partner an orgasm — yet again.

- ashamed to tell your partner what you really want to do in bed.

But guess what?

So is someone else.

Sexual anxiety isn't new and it isn't unique. Most of us are affected or have been affected by some degree of sexual insecurity. It comes with being human. Sometimes it feels like it's only you because those conversations are generally avoided, and not surprisingly so.

It's uncomfortable. It's embarrassing. You feel weird just imagining yourself telling someone about it. And you know what? It's probably not your fault.

Whatever anxieties you have, what's not okay is doing nothing about them.

Don't hide from your anxieties. This can lead to worse feelings in the future. There's a saying that goes something like, "What you repress only grows stronger." If we flip that around, we can say, "What you express loses power over you."

One of the best ways I've found to work through these anxieties and insecurities is to talk about them. I know that sounds like advice that's given to everyone about everything that bothers people.

But I seriously believe that these specific anxieties are best handled externally. Talk about them with a close friend. Let them out of your mind and into the open where someone else can provide a new perspective for you.

Most importantly, talk about them with the person (or people) whom you're experiencing them with – your partner(s). Let them know what's bothering you so they can reassure and help you through it.

It will take some time and some mental effort to recognize insecure, anxious thoughts and work through them, to fully understand your value in the bedroom. But once that happens, you will have set yourself up for some exciting sexual adventures.

It's also important to constantly remind yourself of the ultimate point of sex.

"Wait a minute, Michael. What's the ultimate point of sex?"

This is an individualistic viewpoint, but disregarding procreation for a moment, this is what I think it is:

- To have fun
- To give and receive pleasure
- To act out your desires
- To express feelings, whether they are spontaneous or a result of veteran love
- To have more fun

I call that the sexual fun sandwich.

Sexual Anxieties And How To Work Through Them

Let's get into some specific anxieties and how to demolish their effects on your sex life.

First, I'm going to talk about general sexual anxieties, and then break them up into body part-specific ones. At the end of each description, I'll include ways to work through them.

(This information is based off research and my own experience overcoming sexual anxieties.)

General Anxieties

Body Image, Especially In Bed-

It's not uncommon for us to have insecurities about our physical appearance. Even if every inch of our body is perfect except for one, that one insecurity could weigh on our mind, especially in sexual situations where we feel the most vulnerable.

Think about it: Other than having sex, our most private areas are covered up the majority of the time we're interacting with people. Any shame we may hold about them can be hidden behind our clothing.

As soon as the clothes come off, those parts of our bodies reach the surface. It can be uncomfortable and lead to thoughts that distract us from enjoying the experience. It can even become so debilitating that we refrain from having sex completely. In this way, we avoid exposing that vulnerability.

If you don't experience any of this yourself, it's important to recognize that other people do. Sometimes a simple, sincere, and genuine compliment about your partner's body can be enough to squander those feelings.

Regardless, if you're feeling anxious about your body, don't rely on your partner to help you feel better. This may work in the short term, but it doesn't lead to any lasting self-comfort.

Being comfortable with your body image is less about your physical appearance and more about being comfortable in your body no matter what it looks like.

When you accept your body for what it is, you relax more in sexual situations without worrying about what your partner is thinking of you. When your mind is relaxed, so is your body, leading to greater feelings of pleasure and a higher likelihood of reaching orgasm.

But with that said, working on your physical appearance can't do any harm and will lead to benefits that extend far beyond your sex life.

Overcoming body image anxiety-

The Men's and Women's Health Big Book of Sex (I know it sounds like a "Birds and the Bees" type of children's book, but it's legitimate) compiles the knowledge of thousands of experts and a huge survey of Men's/Women's Health readers.

It's based off hundreds of interviews with some of the most esteemed doctors and researchers in the world, and extensive work reviewing scholarly journals and studies.

Thousands of people responded to *The Big Book of Sex* survey, and contributors include the likes of professors, psychologists, anthropologists, directors of sexual and gender-specific health and wellness centers, relationship advisors, sexologists, sex researchers, and more.

It's pretty comprehensive, and I'll be citing it throughout this chapter.

However, *The Big Book of Sex* was published in 2011, so depending on when you're reading this, it may not be up to date. The advice still holds but the statistics may have changed.

Also, the numbers should not be taken as representative of the entire population, but should be used to gain a general idea. Always use your own judgment when making decisions.

Three ways the book lists to improve body confidence:

Eat healthy food. Overall, your body will feel better and you'll have more energy to devote to sexual activity. It also states that your psyche will benefit from taking control of your health.

Not to mention, healthy eating is far easier than many people claim it to be. Rather than calculating what you put into your body, start by cutting out what you don't want in your body, i.e. fast food, candy, fried foods, sugary foods, etc. Build up a habit of eating healthily first and don't pressure yourself to follow a strict plan.

Once the habit has developed and unhealthy food looks much less appetizing, then look into dietary options that will help you get to the body you want. It takes effort, physically and mentally, but it's worthwhile. Your sex life will thank you, and so will your overall health.

Exercise. A no brainer for anyone, in my opinion. Exercise should be an integral part of everyone's life. Simply putting in the work and seeing your first results will help your body image.

From there, the snowball effect will take over. If the gym isn't your style, tons of other options exist. Go for hikes, play sports, ride your bike around the neighborhood. Some exercise is always better than none.

Take care of the little details. This involves the details of your appearance that by themselves are relatively unremarkable, but together make you feel much better about yourself. And they can be changed in an instant.

This means trimming beards, shaving legs, cutting nails, putting on nail polish, trimming ear and nose hair, brushing and flossing regularly, styling your hair, picking out eye boogers, trimming the fro-down-low; all the minute adjustments that can make you feel more attractive.

But that's enough of the physical stuff. I always try to suggest internal ways of dealing with our issues, because the mind is where these issues are the strongest. If we can solve them at the source, it makes it much easier to handle them on the outside.

Realize that no one cares about how you look as much as you do.

I'm a huge culprit of this too, but sorry, none of us are *that* important that everyone who walks by is judging us. When you see someone and imagine them judging your body, they are most likely imagining you judging there's as well, no matter how great they look.

When you are in bed with someone and you're worrying about what your partner is thinking, realize they could be worrying about what you're thinking as well. It's two-sided.

So stop placing so much value on the appearance of you or your partner, and place more value on how you feel with each other, the passion of the sex, what moves you can try that you've never done before, how you can play around with the balance of dominance. These are just a few aspects of sex we have discussed so far that can make it so dynamic.

Poor body image can be a major struggle for many people in their sex lives, but it's largely in our minds, and that's good news. Recognizing those thoughts and consciously eliminating them, combined with living a healthy lifestyle, will leave you feeling more comfortable exposing your vulnerability and open the doors to sexual experiences you never dreamed you would have.

Not Being Able to Pleasure Your Partner Or Give Them An Orgasm-

For me, being able to pleasure my partner is a huge deal. If I wasn't able to (and I've had partners where this was the case) I'd feel terrible about myself. You start questioning what you did wrong, if it's your body, if you have no control over it, or if there's something else you should have done.

The fact of the matter is: Everyone's body is different. Some people orgasm easier than others. Some people feel more or less pleasure than others.

Often, whether you can pleasure them is less about you alone but rather about your *compatibility* together; physically, emotionally, and mentally.

It could also be your partner. If they've never had an orgasm before or they've only had a few, then their body may not recognize how to progress through each stage leading to climax. Their genitals could also be more desensitized than average.

However, you are not off the hook. You have lots of techniques at your disposal to give your partner more pleasure and increase the likelihood of them reaching an orgasm (however, it must be noted that having an orgasm should not be the ultimate goal. It's definitely a good goal, but it shouldn't take excessive priority).

Once you have some weapons in your arsenal to bust out, your anxiety should almost completely go away.

Pleasuring your partner-

After reading this guide, read some books to further your knowledge. That's what I did and it did wonders for my sex life. Here are a couple I suggest:

- *The Men's and Women's Health Big Book of Sex*
- *She Comes First – The Thinking Man's Guide To Pleasuring A Woman,* by Ian Kerner, Ph. D.

Within these two books you'll find a vast wealth of sexual knowledge.

The Big Book of Sex gives you a great overview of sex and the many different aspects, including how your own body functions, your partner's body functions, workouts and diets to get you in sexual shape, understanding the opposite sex, STIs (sexually transmitted infections), sexual anxieties and health concerns, birth control, making passion last in long term relationships, and much more.

If you have a vagina and/or are not interested in giving pleasure to those who have vaginas, you may see no point in reading *She Comes First*. I know that if I saw a book about how to pleasure people with penises I wouldn't put forth any effort to read it. But, I am going to make an argument:

As I said before, the author could have easily made the book gender neutral. In addition, and this goes for everyone, understanding your body and how you reach the heights of pleasure is one of the best ways for your partner to understand it.

Huh? What? Why?

Because you can give them advice on how to pleasure you best.

The more you understand about your own body, the better equipped your partner will be.

You can also try watching your partner pleasure themselves. This will show you where they like to be touched, how they like to be rubbed, the right pace, and what gets them over that final hump to orgasmic release.

There is no single way to give everyone an orgasm. Everybody reaches orgasm differently and experiences pleasure differently.

What's the tried and true way to learn how to pleasure your partner?

Ask them.

Getting An STI or The Possibility Of Receiving One From A Recent Partner-

I've had a couple STI scares, and they are terrifying. There were times when I wished I could go back to being a virgin rather than experience the possibility of having an STI.

The possibility of getting a sexually transmitted infection is absolutely not worth having unsafe sex. And I'm sure actually having one is 100,000% not worth it. It's a serious health concern that every sexually active and future sexually active person should be aware of.

That being said, here's what I suggest:

- Get tested at least every two partners.

- Always have a couple condoms on you when you go out, regardless of gender or sexual orientation, and especially if you plan on engaging in anal play.

- If you are using a condom, *always put the damn condom on or have your partner put the damn condom on*. There is no use in having it with you if you are not going to use it, and there is nothing worse than waking up in the morning after a night of unprotected sex, wrought with anxiety about the myriad of STIs you may have just caught. It's just not worth it. Trust me.

In my view, the possibility of getting an STI should not lead you to completely refrain from sexual activity. But remember, you must always use your own best judgment, especially when your health is concerned.

For Those With Penises

Penis size-

As I mentioned before, I've experienced this anxiety (actually, I've experienced almost all of these anxieties to some degree).

Personally, I blew it out of proportion, and if you're experiencing it I'm sure you are too.

Overcoming it-

The Big Book of Sex states that the average length of an erect penis is 5.1 inches, and that "if your erection measures 4 to 6 inches, you're quite normal."

So how should you truly measure your penis?

One: If you are with a partner who only cares about your size, then you're with the wrong partner (or partners).

Two: Your penis is not the only value you have in the bedroom, by far. Read the books I listed above about pleasuring your partner, especially *She Comes First*.

The author went through his own struggles with sexual anxiety (namely premature ejaculation), learned how he could pleasure his partner in other ways, and eventually became a sex therapist.

With the wealth of knowledge out there, there's no reason why you can't follow the same type of path.

Three: There's an advertising principle called "Length Implies Strength." It's related to the length of your ad and sales copy and how it communicates the credibility of the words. Luckily for many people, this principle is not as sound when it comes to their size.

While length can be a huge turn on for partners, girth may actually be the measurement that's really providing most of the pleasure. For those that don't know what girth is, here's a definition:

Girth – the size of someone or something measured around the middle (Merriam-Webster)

Basically, it's the circumference of your penis.

Here's an excerpt taken from She Comes First describing the anatomy of the vagina:

"Rare is the man who says, "I made love to her as subtly and lightly as a feather"; "I grazed her vulva as with the delicate wings of a butterfly"; "I barely touched her she came so hard!" And yet such language would be more appropriate, as the inner two thirds of the vagina are substantially less sensitive than the outer third."

Once you enter the vagina, most of the nerve endings (which provide the pleasure) are in the first couple inches or so. The same is true of the anus. The G-Spot and prostate are located a couple inches into their respective genitals.

Strictly in terms of pleasure, the clitoris, outer and inner lips, vaginal entrance, and the first third of the vagina are where most of the pleasure is happening.

The author, Ian Kerner, argues that society is too fixated on the power of the penis in providing pleasure, when we should be focusing our efforts on creating "pleasure not just with our penises, but with our hands and mouths, bodies and minds."

My point isn't to undermine the importance of your member. It's to show that it's not your only value. I'm not doing the book justice, so I highly recommend buying it and reading it yourself.

All of the previous information in this guide should be a testament to why it is not your only value as well.

Just like anything, if you are basing your self-worth on something external, like the size of your penis, you are only making your identity more vulnerable to outside forces.

So, reorient your sexual self-worth to other aspects of sex, such as oral sex, teasing, foreplay, multitasking, and the balance of dominance, and gradually over time you will overcome your anxiety.

Premature Ejaculation-

Premature ejaculation occurs when someone with a penis climaxes too early during sexual intercourse.

My experience with premature ejaculation has been somewhat sporadic. When it happens too quickly, it's usually because it's been a long time since I last had sex or because I haven't masturbated in a while.

Either way, it sucks. But it's not as huge of a deal as you could be making it out to be, and tons of ways exist to overcome it.

Overcoming Premature Ejaculation-

The Men's and Women's Health book lists many ways to last longer, but I'm going lay mine out first, because it's my book and I can do what I want:

- **Have more sex.** If this is possible for you, have as much sex as you can. Get your penis accustomed to the feeling of sexual activity. If you come early the first time, take a 15-30 minute break until you're ready to go again (the refractory period), then try again. See if you last longer. Typically, you will last longer if you have already ejaculated.
- **When you're having sex and you feel yourself reaching the point of no return, pull out immediately and let**

yourself readjust. However, don't just stop the interaction entirely. Even if you are out of action for a bit, keep your partner in the action with oral sex, finger play, manual stimulation, or using a toy until you are ready to go again.

- **Try different positions.** For instance, doggy style positions provide less stimulation than missionary. If you feel like you're about to come, you can switch positions and use that transition time to take a short break (don't forget The Art of the Transition!)

- **Try not to mentally focus so much on how your penis feels.** Keep the motion going, but pay attention to touching your partner's body, kissing them, their hands grabbing your arm – something else that's going on. Distract yourself from the feeling of your penis.

Take it away Men's and Women's Health:

- **Start-stop.** Try to develop a strong intuition for when you're about to climax. When you feel it coming, stop all of your motion and take a short break.

- **This method physically cuts off the urge to ejaculate:** Once you feel you're about to come, "you or your partner squeezes the head of your penis with a thumb and index finger to thwart ejaculation. Squeeze right below the head, focusing the pressure on the urethra – the tube running along the underside of the penis. This pushes blood out of the penis and momentarily represses the ejaculatory response." Once you can do this on command, you can train yourself to last longer. Try practicing while masturbating as well.

- **Have a pre-sex orgasm.** If you know you're going to have sex soon, masturbate.

- **Use a numbing condom.** Benzocaine, a topical anesthetic that reduces sensation in your penis, is used in some condoms, such as Trojan Extended Pleasure and Durex Performax. Keep the condom on, because if the anesthetic leaks out it could numb your partner. You can also use anesthetic gel designed for teething infants or gum inflammation. However, on the same note, be sure all of the gel is absorbed, or put a condom on, so you don't numb your partner.

- **Have your partner be on top.**

- **Give your partner an orgasm first.** This will take some of the pressure off.

- **Stop thinking about your orgasm.** Whether you're thinking about having an orgasm or trying to stop yourself, you are still using the part of your brain responsible for triggering an orgasm. Focus on something else, like gently pulling your partner's hair, kissing them, or sucking on their neck.

With all of these techniques, don't be hesitant to ask your partner to help you out. Odds are, they'll be more than happy to help you overcome any anxieties you have, just like you should be for them.

Erectile Dysfunction-

This is one anxiety that had quite a lasting impact on me. Not so much that it happened often, but that I was always worried it would happen.

ED, or erectile dysfunction, is the inability to gain or maintain an erection.

It has only happened to me when I've been too drunk. But especially when I was about to have sex sober, I'd imagine it happening and I'd worry about not being able to get it up.

The funny thing was, it never actually happened, but I still worried about it. Just goes to show how much of this stuff can truly be in your head.

Overcoming Erectile Dysfunction-

There's a prevailing feeling that if you can't get it up even one time, you become less sexually valuable, at least in your own mind.

You're not any less sexually valuable. Your body has simply betrayed you, and it's not that you don't find your partner attractive or that you're not turned on. It's largely out of your control. If you *would* get it up if you could, then you have nothing to feel bad about.

But you *can* adjust your lifestyle to help you out.

A large part of ED has to do with your health. Here's what *The Big Book of Sex* has to say (neglecting taking pills, as you should solely consult your doctor for that):

- **Eat dark fruits**. Dark fruits, like blackberries, blueberries, and bilberries, have anthocyanins, which are "ultrapowerful antioxidants that attack the free radicals present in our bloodstream. When too many free radicals are present in your bloodstream, nitric oxide goes down – and so does your penis." Nitric oxide is crucial for good blood flow.

- **Quit smoking**. Another benefit of quitting smoking, other than living longer and reducing the risk of cancer, is better sex.

- **Manage your stress**. Easier said than done, but high levels of stress stimulate production of epinephrine, a type of adrenaline that messes with your arteries. It causes the arteries to harden — restricting blood flow. Experts suggest focusing on what is happening in the present rather than dwelling on stressful thoughts, to help alleviate some of this stress. The same advice can be applied in the bedroom. Absorb yourself in the sexuality and let your mind go.

- **Lose weight**. Losing weight lowers your body's overall estrogen levels.

For Those With Vaginas

Not Reaching Orgasm-

The book states that on average, it typically takes women (and I'm guessing, all people with vaginas) longer to orgasm than men (or those with penises). The book says it's 2.6 minutes for men versus 27 minutes for women.

This creates a legitimate concern. First, they're worried they may miss out on the extraordinary release felt during orgasm. Second, they may feel that if they don't orgasm, then their partner will feel bad about themselves.

Neither of these sound like attractive outcomes, so what's someone with a vagina to do?

Overcoming this anxiety-

First, get to know your body. If you don't know how you best climax, it's hard to let your partner know the best way to do it. This means masturbating and experimenting.

Try toys, try thinking about different fantasies, try using lube, not using lube; there are lots of options. Find out which one or ones work best for you.

And don't be afraid to give your partner advice in bed. They should be more than enthusiastic to follow it, because they should want you to orgasm as well.

Also, this is going to sound weird to some of you, but if you feel a sensation like you're about to pee, let it come – literally.

Especially with G-Spot orgasms, the sensation to pee is a common feeling. As Ian Kerner notes in She Comes First, "the G-spot generally responds to a more persistent, massaging pressure. It's not uncommon for a woman [*or those with a vagina*] to feel a fleeting urge to urinate when this area is stimulated."

Those of you who have heard of, seen, or experienced squirting orgasms know what I'm talking about here. Don't deprive yourself by holding back if you feel like you need to pee. You may be on the verge of having an amazing orgasm.

You may have also heard of kegel exercises. If not, the "Kegel" is a muscle in the pelvic floor, named after Dr. Arnold Kegel, who observed that this is one of the prominent muscles that contract during orgasm. He then came up with a number of exercises to strengthen these muscles, resulting in increased pleasure.

If you're still curious which muscle this is specifically, pretend like you are trying to stop yourself from peeing. Do it. Right now.

That's your kegel muscle. Ian Kerner notes that doing these exercises regularly can increase the quality of orgasmic contractions.

A few more techniques to try:

- Just like people who experience erectile dysfunction, those with vaginas can also try giving themselves an orgasm just before having sex. Except, when they have already had an orgasm it becomes easier, rather than harder, for them to have subsequent ones.

- Use a vibrator while having sex to add extra stimulation. The clitoris is said to be the epicenter of all pleasure for those with vaginas.

- Finally, don't be shy about taking care of yourself if your partner is done (assuming they don't want to help you). However, don't do it out of spite. Let them know that it's not about them, and if they'd like to help you out, they are more than welcome to. And more than likely, they will be happy to help you climax as well.

Distracting Thoughts While Having Sex-

This isn't necessarily a sexual "anxiety" per say, but it's important so I want to touch on it.

Here are some stats from the Men's and Women's Health survey regarding what thoughts can be distracting women (or anyone) while having sex:

- Their weight: 26%
- They won't orgasm: 20%
- Other parts of their body: 17%
- Their partner isn't enjoying it: 14%
- Someone might walk in: 9%
- Falling pregnant: 5%
- Other (getting an STI, being used by their partner for sex, their partner doesn't respect them, their partner might not orgasm): 9%

That's 10 different worries possibly weighing on someone's mind at any one time, while trying to enjoy the sexual experience.

This goes for anyone: Being stuck inside your head is one of the worst hindrances to enjoying sex. Cut out your thinking as much as possible. Maybe even practice meditation.

When you are thinking about other stuff, you are not relaxed and you're not focused on the pleasure your body is experiencing. Try to be as natural as possible. Get into a sexual zone where you feel as though your movements are happening automatically. Focus on your partner. Focus on the passion.

Recognize when other thoughts pop into your head and destroy them as fast as possible. The best way to do this is to change something up quickly.

Kiss your partner. Try changing positions. Go grab a toy or some lube. Put a blindfold on. Distract yourself from your distracting thoughts and stay in the moment.

The more you practice having sex while shutting off your thoughts, the more you'll develop sexual intuition, where you'll intuitively and instinctively progress through sex, almost as if you're in a trance. You'll come out of it saying,

"Whoa... What just happened? That was amazing!"

Becoming Pregnant-

Many STIs are easily identifiable and treatable within a matter of hours, days, or weeks.

Now, I'm not calling pregnancy an STI, but it can be an unwanted consequence of having sex, leading to 18 years (or more) of financial, emotional, and life commitment. It can be a life changer, and not an ideal one, for you or the child coming into the World. Hence, the term "unwanted."

It's a real concern. And since it is those with vaginas who hold the ultimate responsibility of nurturing the baby within their body, it's much more of a concern for them than it is for people with penises (despite it being a huge concern for any gender).

The first order of business is to use a condom every time you have sex. This will calm your mind down immensely. Next, consider getting on birth control.

The Big Book of Sex has an entire guide listing 17 different kinds of birth control; popular brands, cost, how to use them, their effectiveness, what each is best for, what each is not recommended for, the risks, potential side effects, whether you need a prescription, when specifically you are protected, and the active ingredients in each. So the information is definitely out there.

(*The Big Book of Sex* should be the textbook for Sex Ed classes.)

Educate yourself and decide if birth control is right for you. Combining birth control and a condom, you've got a double whammy of peace of mind and a much lower likelihood of becoming pregnant.

Closing Thoughts on Sexual Anxieties and Insecurities

Sex is an amazing part of life, and one that should be experienced to its fullest. Unfortunately, it comes with a lot of doubt, anxiety, insecurity, and misconception.

Hopefully I dispelled some of it in this section. I know this is not an exhaustive list of sexual anxieties, and I still experience my own sexual anxiety, but to a much smaller degree than I used to. This is part of what makes my sex life fulfilling, and what I believe can help you do the same.

Moving on to a crucially important topic for navigating your sex life.

What are your sexual values?

Chapter 17

WHAT ARE YOUR SEXUAL VALUES?

In any aspect of life, our values help us decide what we choose to accept into our lives and what we choose to reject.

Sometimes this happens consciously, and sometimes it happens unbeknownst to the individual.

I think dating provides a good example of this. Your values determine much of who you date, and they pop up constantly.

Imagine you are a devout follower of your faith and you meet an awesome person. This person makes you laugh, they are fun to be around, you find them attractive, they get along with all of your friends, etc.

Then you find out they are 100% atheist. In your mind, you have always pictured yourself ending up with someone who may not have to follow your specific religion, but who devotes themselves to some sort of religion. This is a big thing for you, and you are almost uncompromising in terms of this trait.

Despite how much you like them, your conflicting values may override your feelings, hindering the possibility of you two dating.

In dating, this type of instance plays out in many ways, such as in differences in values regarding one's profession, their health, their life ambition, their goals, their current stage in life, what they are looking for in a relationship, etc.

These values act as natural filters for your dating life, filtering in the people who are right for you and filtering out the people who are not.

I first heard about this concept from Mark Manson. I realized the same thing applies to our sex lives, so I have adapted it to our discussion.

Whether you realize it or not, you value certain aspects of sex. When you meet someone with conflicting values to your own, or you end up in bed with someone with conflicting values to your own, odds are the interaction won't go any further.

You may meet someone, find them attractive, connect with them, and go home with them that night. But once you have sex, you find that the individual is a selfish lover who doesn't have any interest in your pleasure.

If you value mutual caring for each other's pleasure when having sex, this becomes a conflicting value, making you unlikely to want to sleep with them again.

As another example, the sex may be really good with someone and you connect on all the right levels. But when it comes time to talk about your sex life and trying new things, your partner shuts off, not opening themselves to discussion whatsoever.

If you value open communication in your sexual relationships, and your partner values avoiding these discussions, this conflicting value may cause a breach in your relationship and your sex life.

Sometimes, people understand that conflicting values are at the root of these types of interactions, but other people are completely unaware of it. Either way, they play a major role in the direction of your sex life.

My point: When you understand the sexual values you hold, you are better equipped to navigate your sex life in the direction YOU want it to go.

When you find someone who doesn't share your values, you can make a better decision about how to handle it. When you find someone who shares your values, you can make better a decision about whether to move forward with them or not.

However, having conflicting values with someone doesn't give you permission to be spiteful or to make them feel bad for not sharing your values. It is simply a state of being and should be left at that. If you part ways it should be on neutral ground, not because one of you feels high and mighty and the other feels guilty for not sharing the other's values.

It's a natural occurrence. It happens all the time. And it should be handled in a mature manner.

That being said, when you do share sexual values with someone, it can be a beautiful thing and lead to some of the best sex of your life.

This is when things just click together. Your sexual flow feels natural. Your communication is open and understanding, and you grow together as sexual beings. It's truly beautiful.

Which Sexual Values Do You Hold?

Let's figure out which sexual values you hold, assuming you are not entirely conscious of them already.

I'm going to list some of the more powerful ones. They will be different for everyone on an individual basis, but I believe this is a good general outline.

Being yourself in the bedroom. You value someone who can be their true selves, even when they are lying completely naked with you. You value someone who you feel comfortable enough around to be your true self as well.

Having fun. This is a big one for me. You value people who can laugh at themselves when they're naked, or look at some mishap afterwards and see the humor in it. Sex shouldn't be serious all the time. For whatever reason, some of the funniest stuff happens when you're having sex.

Mutually caring about each other's pleasure. This is when two people take an active interest in pleasuring each other. The scale of who-is-pleasuring-who is relatively balanced, and when it becomes too unbalanced, the partners work together to take steps to rectify it.

Being open and honest. You value people who will tell you straight up what's going on in their mind, rather than bottling up what they are frustrated about. You also value this in yourself, and try your best to hold yourself to it.

Communication. You value being able to discuss certain aspects of sex in an open environment that is free of judgment.

You also value being able to talk about issues in a way that doesn't hurt the other person's feelings.

Safety. You value being safe in the bedroom, both by practicing proper hygiene and protecting against STIs and unwanted pregnancy. You also value being in a safe environment where you can be vulnerable with another person.

Trust. Trusting each other is huge when it comes to having great sex. You need to be able to trust that your partner will keep certain things about your sex life a secret if you ask them to. They should be able to trust you as well.

Comfort. You value being comfortable around someone. This means that when things get awkward (which is practically inevitable, especially in the beginning) you two will be able to work through it and make it into something positive. You also feel comfortable being naked around them and expressing your desires to them.

Connection. Sex is an intimate act, even if it is only for one night. I have always valued the connection that I make with someone, in committed or uncommitted relationships. It makes sex deeper and more fulfilling.

Status. You may value the status of your partner in the bedroom. At first, many will see this as the superficial aspects, such as their looks. We can also look beyond that to how cool they are, how well-rounded their personality is, how sociable they are, etc.

Sexual compatibility. This is how well you two match together on a sexual level. Does your flow coincide? Do you have a good balance of dominance and submission? Do you fit together on both a physical and mental level?

These are just some of the values you may have in the bedroom. Try your best to delve deeper into the reasons why you like certain people or certain things in bed, and you may end up finding that the root cause is from what you value.

Once you know what you value, you will be able to communicate this to your partner or partners, and you will be able to screen for the people who will be your most fulfilling sexual partners.

Chapter 18

SEXUAL COMPATIBILITY

I have discussed sexual compatibility quite a lot, so I will keep this chapter short.

When my partner and I first got together, we immediately knew that we were sexually compatible. Everything just clicked.

Our minds worked the same in the bedroom. We hardly had to say anything about actually having sex, because most of it happened naturally. There was a natural sexual connection between us that was hard to explain at the time.

All we knew was we were sexually compatible, and it was awesome.

Sexual compatibility can be something that you intuitively feel, like between my partner and I. But I believe it can also be raised and nurtured.

If your sex life isn't so great, take responsibility for it. Don't blame someone else for bad sex. It doesn't help and it only makes people feel bad about themselves.

If you take responsibility for it, you can do your research and help out a partner who may need to brush up their skills. You can also initiate more communication about your desires, write up some lists and trade them like we learned in the communication chapter, and lead you and your partner towards a better sex life.

Working to grow together like this will nurture sexual compatibility. You will foster a stronger connection, deepen your sexual knowledge together, and it will materialize in the bedroom.

The more you understand about sexuality, and about your own body, the more likely you will be sexually compatible with the partners that enter your life.

Chapter 19

A NOTE ABOUT PORN

As I said before, I watched a lot of porn in my pubescent days. I don't necessarily regret it, because porn answered a lot of my questions about sexuality when I was that age. However, I do believe there are much healthier ways I could have found those answers.

Porn is not reality. Porn is a business, and their business is to make sales and increase profit, just like any other.

The way they do that is by appealing to our deepest desires for control and intimacy. They appeal to our desire to live out our fantasies vicariously through the people on the screen, without having to face some of the tough realities of real life.

They do this by using certain angles that make things look bigger. They use actors that have undergone plastic surgery to accentuate their body parts. They use "buffers" to help people maintain erections. And they fake orgasms for the camera.

I am not denouncing the industry. I am warning you that you should not take too much of what you see in porn as reality, as I did when I was younger. It leads to a lot of unnecessary stress and anxiety, and it also portrays an unrealistic perception of what sex is like in real life and what it truly means.

Rather than living vicariously through porn, try your best to make your fantasies into a real reality. Often times, it starts by working on yourself – by getting your lifestyle in order, by increasing your sexual knowledge, by taking an interest in your health and wellness, by building a fulfilling social circle, by expressing yourself freely to people, by finding a passion that will carry you through your life.

After that, sex will come naturally to you, and you will wonder why you spent so much time watching porn when you could have been experiencing something much more meaningful first hand.

I've found that porn in small doses is not detrimental. When it becomes a borderline addiction, or a full-fledged addiction, that's when it has adverse effects on your life.

If you watch porn, know that the real thing is much, much better, and is fully attainable.

Chapter 20

THE SEXUAL CONQUEST

Sex is such an interesting part of our lives. We can become completely different people once we sneak under the sheets with someone.

There is so much to explore, so many parts of our human psyche that are still untapped, waiting for the right key to come unlock them.

I believe that almost anyone can be consumed by the allure sex poses. It becomes a challenge to reach certain milestones – losing your virginity, receiving your first oral sex, giving your first oral sex, having sex in public for the first time, trying your first sex toy, making love for the first time.

It's fun. There's also a certain amount of ego involved. It feels good to be doing this stuff, and I do think that sex is a fundamental need we have as human beings.

But it's also important not to place too much emphasis on your "success" or "failure" in this conquest. I've been through periods where I wasn't having any sex, and for whatever reason, I let it affect my self-esteem and my sense of self-worth.

This is an unhealthy view of sexuality. You are letting your mind become vulnerable to an outside force that can be largely out of your control.

The conquest shouldn't be a conquest at all. There shouldn't be anything to conquer, or to do better than someone else, or to do before someone else.

It should be an exploration of this aspect of life. You should try your best to seek the truth in your sex life. Find out what you truly want. Find a partner or partners who share your desires. Make the most of those experiences.

Don't do this for personal gain or to make yourself feel better. Don't do it to selfishly "get yourself off."

Do it to genuinely share a unique connection with someone.

Do it to have the most fun you possibly can.

I mean, that's what this is all about right? Having a good time?

So take what you have learned here, go forth in your sex life with confidence and determination to find that truth which only you can find, and I will leave you with one last thing:

This may be *The Guide to Great Sex*, but in reality, you are your own guide to great sex.

Navigate wisely.

REFERENCES and FURTHER READING

The Men's and Women's Health Big Book of Sex

She Comes First – *The Thinking Man's Guide to Pleasuring a Woman* - Ian Kerner, Ph. D.

WebMD – The Sexual Response Cycle

Wikipedia – Anal Sex

WebMD – Anal Sex Health Concerns

Wikipedia – Sex Positions

Down to Earth Guide to STIs – Mark Manson